Cystitis

How to Prevent Infection and Inflammation

Angela Kilmartin

Thorsons
An Imprint of HarperCollins*Publishers*

With abiding thanks to the inspirational works
of Philip and Florence

Thorsons
An Imprint of HarperCollins*Publishers*
77–85 Fulham Palace Road,
Hammersmith, London W6 8JB
1160 Battery Street,
San Francisco, California 94111–1213

Published by Thorsons 1994

10 9 8 7 6 5 4 3

© Angela Kilmartin 1994

Angela Kilmartin asserts the moral right to
be identified as the author of this work

A catalogue record for this book
is available from the British Library

ISBN 0 7225 2996 1

Printed and bound in Great Britain by
Caledonian International Book Manufacturing, Glasgow

CONTENTS

PREFACE

I lost my honeymoon, all my holidays, my operatic career and my marriage directly or indirectly because of recurrent cystitis. It is my avowed aim never to let another woman suffer unnecessarily from cystitis.

Every year on 8th August I recall the anniversary of my first attack, two days into my honeymoon. I was incontinent, feverish, passing bloody urine, screaming, fainting from the pain and frightened to death. It remains one of my life's most anguished memories.

From then until 1972 I had 78 such attacks, all treated with antibiotics or operations. Thrush from the antibiotics caused equal misery, but nothing was offered to stop the attacks from starting in the first place. I now know for sure that prevention alone is the key to freedom from the pain, misery and stress caused by cystitis.

Unable to guarantee stage appearances, I was forced to abandon a promising career in opera and instead decided to take revenge upon cystitis. In 1971 I founded the U & I (Urinary Infection/You & I) Club and a magazine specifically for cystitis victims. Unfortunately I had to fold the magazine in 1981 when I went abroad for a long time and the Club has since disbanded. This is the sixth book I have written about cystitis. Many campaigns followed the publication of my first books – a Health Education Council leaflet, a film, TV and radio programmes, a book written for the US market, medical lectures, a video and much more.

I have been free of trouble since 1976, when correct prevention routines were finally instituted. To date, millions of other sufferers the world over have been helped or completely cured as a result of my work. I hope this book will help you, too, to be rid once and for all of cystitis.

FOREWORD

Cystitis is a bane of womankind. From its mildest form of irritation to the severe disease of a life-threatening illness, cystitis has been with us for many centuries. Like other commonly occurring conditions, it has perhaps been put a little to one side by formal medicine; doctors hand out a pocketful of antibiotics and a bit of advice on extra fluids. It was not until Angela Kilmartin started her pioneering work on actually identifying the details of this disease that it came into a medical spotlight.

This book outlines the work she has done for many years to help women with cystitis. It is an excellent account of the background science of the subject and gives very good advice to those who have it. More importantly, perhaps, it advises people on how to prevent cystitis. There is also a very important section on non-bacterial cystitis, for this is a mystery still to some doctors. Angela Kilmartin again dissects the problem and gives first-rate advice on its management. This book is a must for any woman who has ever had the miseries of a urine infection. It is well produced and will help women. I recommend it thoroughly.

Geoffrey Chamberlain, President
Royal College of Obstetricians and Gynaecologists, London
March 1994

Part 1
BACTERIAL CYSTITIS

Chapter 1
HELP!

Bacterial cystitis is caused by germs invading the bladder; that is why it is also known as a urinary infection. The first half of this book will help you to stop it! Consider it your first positive step on the road to recovery for good and all. Say farewell to courses of debilitating antibiotics and their wretched accompaniment, vaginal thrush. This book will show you how to prevent, simply, quickly and from today, what could otherwise be a life-long problem with bacterial cystitis.

Cystitis is a Greek word, probably first coined on the Greek island of Kos. On that lovely island was the world's first medical school, now in glorious ruin but still visited by thousands each year. It stretches from the base of a steeply sloping hill to its peak and was founded *circa* 500 BC by Hippocrates – he of the Hippocratic Oath by which he bound all the first doctors whom he trained at the school.

If you ever visit this ancient site, take note of the levels of the hill on which the hospital was built. Each level of the hill (and the hospital) corresponded to a section of the trunk of the human body. The bowels, bladder and genital departments were dug out below the base of the hill into the ground. The very top of the hill was the home of the department of psychi-

3

atry! To this day, teaching hospitals put the VD unit either on ground level or below!

Cyst is Greek for a pouch or sac or bladder; *itis* means inflammation which may or may not be caused by infection. About 60 per cent of all cystitis patients have an infection, that is, named bacteria in the urine sample. I had that, too. It was this infection in my urethra and bladder that rocked my young marriage to its core. My husband worried so much that he had caused my cystitis that he went with another woman to see if she would 'catch' it from him. I never knew of this for years and, when he told me, I felt so sorry for him because it showed how desperate he was to find some kind of answer to our problem. For five years I suffered attacks of urinary infection every two to three weeks, and they doubled in misery once permanent vaginal thrush had set in, knocking the stuffing out of our love and our limits of patient endurance.

We did survive it, but in later years we seemed 'jinxed' by marital difficulty and unable to pull ourselves together. I believe we used up a mountain of good will, kindness and perseverance fighting my cystitis in those early years, far more than most young marrieds have to face.

Nor did the thrush abate. Nothing was known about how to treat it in the early 1970s except for pessaries and short courses of Nystatin oral tablets (Nystatin is sold as Mycostatin in the US and Australia). There seemed nothing to touch the unremitting candidiasis that had invaded my whole system and kept my vagina sore, red, itchy and full of discharge. Such a vagina could not tolerate sexual intercourse.

So, you see, apart from being very knowledgeable on the help available for sufferers from urinary infections, I know all about the personal social consequences of the suffering. My revenge on it is to write about it and to beat it for you as I did for myself and for the countless women the world over who have followed my advice. Consider this book your first positive step on the road to recovery for good and all. Say farewell to courses of debilitating antibiotics and their wretched accompaniment of vaginal thrush. This book will show you simply and quickly how to prevent, *from today*, what could be a life-long problem with bacterial cystitis.

The kind of help that I offer for sufferers from urinary infections is *preventive* help. How much sooner would you rather prevent the dreaded twinges which signal the onset of yet another attack? Of course, this book also include first aid for helping to get rid of an attack, but that, to my way of thinking, spells failure; failure to stop that attack from ever having started in the first place. It is much more clever to prevent it and to prevent it for good.

Stopping attacks has very beneficial effects all round:

1. You do not need to take further courses of antibiotics.
2. You save a huge amount of money by not having to buy these antibiotics.
3. Trips to the doctor for the condition may cease altogether: no more agonies in the waiting room or difficulties in getting to the surgery.
4. Long-term trouble for the immune system is halted.
5. No further risks of vaginal thrush or candidiasis.
6. Intercourse can be safely and happily enjoyed.
7. Your partner can no longer use this excuse to 'stray'.
8. You can go to work regularly – not have a week off every time you suffer an attack.
8. You can guarantee to do the weekly shopping trip.
9. Fear of future attacks disappears altogether.

Take it from me, preventing trouble is not only easy and cheap, it is also pure bliss to be free of the symptoms.

The Symptoms

The classic symptoms of urinary infection are:

- pain when you pass urine
- frequency of urination and the urgent need to go
- bleeding from the urethral tube as you pass urine
- backache
- fever or raised temperature
- smelly urine

These symptoms present in variable forms. The pain, for instance, starts as a shivery twinge as you finish passing urine on a seemingly ordinary visit to the loo. That shivery twinge sends a cold, upward ripple of sensation in the urethral tube. If steps to abort it are not taken straight away, these twinges progress quite quickly to the scalding, and on to the pain, and further on to what I always describe as the 'scalpel' stage. 'Broken glass' is another common description of the intensely sharp and excruciating pain that accompanies the advanced stage of infection.

Now let's look at a few of these symptoms in more detail

Frequency and Urgency

Do I know about this! In my early attacks I sometimes did not 'make it' to the loo. When this urgency strikes there is absolutely no question of 'holding it': that urine has a will of its own and you leave the close vicinity of a bathroom at your peril! The very delicate mechanisms of bladder and urethral action are thrown into top gear in a desperate attempt to flush the invading bacteria out. It is a defence system that becomes automatic once the invasion signals are sent out.

It works the same way if a food or drink has an allergic effect, or if a chemical upsets the sensitive vulval skin. These non-bacterial causes are discussed in later chapters of this book.

Bleeding

This is a particularly horrible symptom, and a definite sign that a severe bacterial invasion is infiltrating the urethral and bladder lining. It happens quickly in women who have had many past attacks and who now bear scars inside their urethra and bladder. The minute scars are weaker than fresh skin and have a diminished ability to repel bacteria. The more scars you acquire, the more likely you will bleed. Once bacteria gain entrance to the bloodstream, *backache* and *fever* will start. You will feel very ill and may start to shake as your kidneys become infected.

This is really dangerous. Too much of this may scar your kidneys for life. The kidneys may become disfigured and lose their smoothness and bean-like shape. The next step could be to lose the use of these two vital organs. Dialysis twice a week would keep you alive but at great cost and with a severe reduction in the quality of life.

I spend time on the phone these days gritting my teeth telling young women that 'Interstitial Cystitis' (IC) is the new medical flavour of the year! Simply put it means 'between' (inter) 'layers' (stitial) 'bladder' (cyst) 'inflammation or infection' (itis) − in other words, 'infection/inflammation of the layers of the bladder'. This is no more or less than chronic cystitis, the term formerly used. But what causes its severity is still beyond medical know-how or treatment.

In the US, so much surgery has been done on women's bladders that they no longer function and, after years of repeated infections and dilations, the trouble is so chronic that they sometimes need removing. Although I have had one book out in the US since 1979, I am not there in person to do publicity and no self-help really exists. The result is that American women have gone from bad to worse by the million. One support group called the Interstitial Foundation has been formed in the US, but there is no help for damage that has already occurred; bladder damage from scarring is beyond repair. If self-help had begun early and surgery prevented, chronic cystitis would not have developed. Fear of litigation keeps urologists talking about this 'new' condition, IC, and prevents the truth from emerging.

We in Britain have not had a similar proliferation (in part because I am here to stop it!) but increasingly doctors are encouraging patients to think in terms of IC to mask their own inabilities. It is all a result of failure and incomprehension on the part of the vast majority of health professionals.

All of this spells out just how much there is to be gained from stopping early attacks on the first twinges. You absolutely must protect your kidneys because you cannot grow new ones. In the process, prevention saves you from most of the misery of the ordinary attack and from a lot of unnecessary expense as well.

Anyone with an ulcerated bladder lining might like to insist that urine samples are cultured for *over two weeks* in case Helicobacter groups of bacteria which are responsible for stomach/duodenal ulcers can be found. There are specific groups of antibiotics to deal with them.

If antibiotics increase bladder pain this may point to a fungal infestation in which case anti-fungal systemic drugs like Sporanox should be prescribed for at least two weeks. If there is some small improvement continue anti-fungal systemic treatment. Bladder urine and biopsies can be tested for Candida if the laboratory is so requested.

In 1923 a Dr Weston Price in Cleveland, Ohio, USA was heavily involved in proving that accepted knowledge of dental

HELP!

treatments was unjustifiable given his profound experiments on rabbits and the thousands of Case Histories that came his way. The two massive volumes into which he collated his thousands of experiments are called: *Volume I – Dental Infections Oral and Systemic Disease, Volume II – Dental Infections and the Degenerative Diseases.*

These two thrilling books are available to dentists from the British Dental Association Library in Wimpole Street, London. The general public may make an appointment to go and view them but the books may not be taken out except by a dentist registered at the BDA. Reprints may also be bought from America via a Mastercard for 180 dollars from The Price Pottinger Foundation, telephone 001-619-574-7763.

In these volumes are to be found causes of every manner of systemic diseases which originate in teeth. There are scores of pages on kidney disease caused by bad teeth and bad dental treatments, in particular Root Canal Therapy which Dr Price asserts, backed up by his experiments, causes this. In one big chapter on kidneys, apart from the huge number of mentions elsewhere, there are two pages on bladder troubles.

Both men and women as victims of dentally focussed bladder troubles are dealt with in this exciting section. Chronic cystitis, i.e. long term pain, infection and frequency may, he claims, be caused by poor dental treatment and jaw infections. He discloses ulcerated bladders in rabbits which had previously been implanted with diseased root-canalled teeth from both men and women who have had some kind of central nervous system disturbance. In so-called Interstitial Cystitis, bladder ulcers appear to be regularly found to reveal a true diagnosis. Unrelieved pain which may indeed emanate from an involvement with the spinal cord could be relieved if the source is looked for in the spinal column or jaws somewhere. That ulcers are the key link may not be coincidental but simply the bladder reflecting the state of jaw ulceration as well.

Those searching for an answer might also look back to

diaries showing commencement of root canal treatment. Systemic reactions in any gland or organ can commence thereafter at any interval. (Please see my book *Dental Poisoning*, unfinished at this time, 1997.) This may be immediately obvious but more likely some months or years later which may account for the current absence in urology or dentistry to find the answer. In any case no-one would be thinking of linking the teeth to the bladder! But it's worth a ponder and Dr Price is quite specific in his books.

It would be worth removing the root canal treatment by full tooth extraction and monitoring the result. If you have several canal treatments or sites of dental inadequacy try contacting Dr George Meinig, 323 East Matillija 110–151 Ojai, California 93023 and read his book called *Root Canal Cover-Up*. There are dental surgeons who specialise in diagnosis and removal of infected teeth, root canals and bone. One or two are here in the UK as word spreads, such as Robert Hemplemann in Chelsea, London SW1, telephone 0171-370-0055, but the leaders are in America. Dr Christopher Hussar in Reno, Nevada is one such. He works on Pan-oral X-rays showing areas of disease which would be overlooked as unremarkable by most dentists. Dr Hussar and Dr Meinig read X-rays with a far more subtle and sophisticated eye. All dentists should attend the update course from the Americans when they come over.

Allow time for bladder ulcers to deplete after any tooth or canal extraction though usually systemic disease or pain elsewhere other than the bladder can resolve exceptionally fast after exctraction. Some people literally throw away there crutches on the journey home from the extraction!

If this is not the cause of the ulceration then perhaps a course of antibiotics or the full treatment now given for duodenal ulcers caused by Helicobacter Pyelori could be tried. This is because there is a group of bacteria known as Bacters which can be found in the bladder if the laboratory is sufficiently sophisticated and able. Citro bacter has been found in a patient of mine using the London Clinic laboratory. Such unusual bacteria may not be tested for in most laboratories, so ask and show this section to the relevant doctors.

Root Canal Treatments promote infection in the dentine tubules and until the colony of bacteria increases or the toxins start to leak into the canal itself, the patient will not become aware. Bacteria are usually Staphlococcus as Dr Price showed but the jaw infections spreading outwards from infected root canal treatments or careless extractions can show mixed anaerobes and aerobes. These will necessitate very heavy courses of mixed antibiotics to control the infection. Its always worth organising samples from these extractions and curettings of jawbone and tissue in case antibiotics and proof are required. Then sensitive antibiotics can be specifically prescribed.

The Urinary System

Figure 1: The urinary system

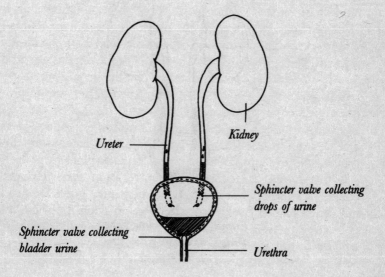

Ureter

Kidney

Sphincter valve collecting drops of urine

Sphincter valve collecting bladder urine

Urethra

Have a look at the diagram of the urinary system shown in Figure 1. The kidneys sift waste body products into liquid and send it down each ureter as urine, until the gentle pressure of several drops on the sphincter valves influences them to open up and allow the urine into the bladder. I have watched this happening during a procedure called a *cystoscopy*, which I was once allowed to view, with the help of a microscope in the *cystoscope* – an instrument with a light for viewing the urethra and bladder. I was thrilled to see this clever little internal activity. It goes on 24 hours a day for as long as you live!

When sufficient urine has collected in the bladder the urethral sphincter bows to pressure and signals to you to go to the lavatory, where you then let it all flow out.

When the urethra is invaded by bacteria, this invasion progresses as shown in Figure 2.

Figure 2: The urethra invaded by bacteria

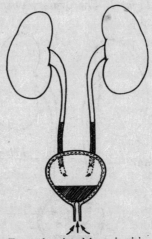

External perianal bacteria rising through out urinary system then into bloodstream

Chapter 2
DON'T CRY!

Curse and swear, yes! But crying usually renders you incapable of any action. Being blinded by tears means you cannot walk round, you cannot get busy to help yourself and it demoralizes you still more. You hunch up over a hankie and feel utterly desperate, as though you have been hit on the head with a brick. Not another one! 'What will Dick think when he gets home and finds me like this again! I can't take any more time off work!', or 'Where can I send the children for the day?', or 'I can't get to the doctor before tonight even if I will be well enough by then; Mum's out for the day so she can't get me anywhere. I just feel so hopeless, so depressed, the pain's getting worse and I'll finish up sitting on the toilet all day.'

The tears pour down, you need another hankie and you start to feel feverish. Every time you pass miserably small amounts of scalding urine, you shiver and yell and cry some more. Then the fear starts, and maybe the bleeding if you have had lots of attacks before. After an hour or so you cannot walk easily, so down onto the carpet you sink, still crying in waves of panic and self-pity. 'Why me?!'

I have been there, reader, I have been there many times and so have countless others. You, in the 90s, are relatively lucky,

. You have this book to read, magazine articles to ⸱⸱⸱ ⸱ through and many doctors who at least mutter about he⸱ping you to help yourself. There was absolutely nothing written or suggested for patients before 1972, when I first started my work and wrote my first articles, after years of suffering with cystitis.

Stop crying – get angry instead. Build up your anger and have a good swear. Once you are up on your feet, go to the kitchen and get busy. Mentally adjust the anger now to productive activity and a wish to fight this rising, intrusive pain and embarrassing frequency. Think yourself lucky it has started at home, that you are not on the bus or the train, or stuck in a traffic jam somewhere!

Think yourself lucky that, as you progress through this book you will learn how to prevent further days like today. Do not give in to it, not now you are going to arm yourself with the best help in the world. It is help that works perfectly and will make such days a thing of the past. Do stop crying, you are going to feel much better in an hour or so!

Practical Steps

What sequence of practical steps should you take when an attack of cystitis begins?

Whenever it starts, no matter what time of day or night, TAKE A URINE SAMPLE BEFORE YOU DO ANY DRINKING.

How to Take a Mid-stream Urine Sample (MSU)
1. Pour boiling water from a kettle into a 1-pint (20 fl. oz/500 ml) heat-proof measuring jug to sterilize it. Just shake it dry and then cover it with a clean cloth until you need it.

2. By the same method, sterilize a small glass jar and lid, if you do not already have a sterile jar from the doctor.
3. Take both to the bathroom and set them down.
4. Still standing up, take two or three wet cotton balls and clean your urethral and vaginal openings.
5. Clean the rim of the lavatory bowl, then sit on this, rather than the seat, so that it is easier to pass the pyrex jug beneath you.
6. Pass a little urine into the lavatory, then catch the midstream in the pyrex jug.
7. Finish the stream into the pan.
8. Clean up, pour the urine sample from the jug into the jar, seal it with the lid.
9. Label the jar with your name, address, the time and your doctor's name.
10. Store this in the fridge for the time being – but get it to the doctor or laboratory quickly.

This is obviously easy to do at home, but if an attack starts when you are at work or out, try to get home – if you are on holiday, get to your hotel bedroom – and get that specimen organized. It should go very quickly to a laboratory via your doctor or a special clinic or a helpful friend. If it has to wait a bit, it *must* be put straight in the fridge.

Go to the doctor if you want and get some antibiotics 'in case', but you may not need to take them.

Mild- and medium-cultured growths of bacteria in the urine sample may be overcome by first aid without having to take debilitating antibiotics which can cause vaginal thrush and more discomfort.

Once you reach home, or your hotel or, of course, at work if you know that you will not be able to make it home in time, proceed as recommended in the sections that follow.

Three Hours of First-aid Management on the First or Second Twinge

CYSTITIS

Having taken the MSU,

1. Drink half a pint (10 fl. oz/250 ml) of water straight away and another half pint every 20 minutes for three hours. No more and no less. If you drink before taking the MSU, the sample will be too diluted to analyse correctly.
2. In that initial half-pint (and repeating on the second and third hour), mix any of the following:

   - 1 level teaspoon of bicarbonate of soda or
   - a sachet of Cymalon or Cystopurin from any pharmacy. Follow packet instructions

3. Take three strong painkillers (such as paracetamol) with another quick glass of water, and a further dose in three hours' time.
4. Fill two hot-water bottles, if you have them. Sit in a comfy chair or go to bed and wedge one bottle at your back, cover the other with a towel and wedge that up between your legs over your vulva.
5. Help the bladder to flush even more by taking a diuretic such as Frusemide, if your doctor will allow you, or by having one strong *coffee cup* full of coffee on the hour every hour for just three hours. Water, anyway, is a good diuretic.

This simple first aid has many advantages:

- The pain is very swiftly reduced.
- Any bleeding will shortly stop.
- By acting fast, bacterial growth rate is halted.
- You can stay at work if you must.
- You will protect your kidneys from permanent scarring.
- There may prove to be no necessity for antibiotics at all.
- It is very cheap!

Once the three hours are up you will be much better. Do

not attempt to change the timing or the dosages; they have been carefully worked out. For instance, extra water will alter your blood-pressure and you may feel dizzy, but with the half-pint every 20 minutes for three hours you should not have any adverse reaction.

The bicarbonate, Cystopurin or Cymalon all act to alkanize the urine so that bacteria, whose preferred environment is mild acidity, cannot thrive. Choose whichever one you like. You are most likely already to have some bicarbonate in the house (with the other cake-baking ingredients?); getting the other two will probably mean a trip to the local pharmacy.

If you hate the bicarbonate in water, try it in a small amount of jam followed by a drink.

After the three hours, keep a half-pint going down about every hour, and tail that off as the situation stabilizes. The painkillers are also very useful in calming the bladder nerve endings and stopping them from unnecessary activity once the bacteria begin to go.

Washing the Perineum

A lot of women ask me whether it is helpful to do any perineal washing in an attack. At this first-aid stage, without the urine sample result, you do not know whether this attack is due to bacterial invasion or something else.

(For this section of the book, dealing solely with infection, I am going to assume that the attack being dealt with is caused by bacterial infection, so I will suggest the following washing. You should understand, though, as you progress through the book, that recurrent urinary infections will soon be a thing of the past because you will learn how to prevent them. I have, therefore, put this first aid early in the book because it may be the last time you need it!)

If we do assume for this once that, in view of previous

attacks which have shown positive bacteria in the urine sample, this attack is probably also due to bacteria, then we may also assume that your whole perineum is, at this moment, running with bacteria. So how to clean it thoroughly?

While you are on the loo, pour some warm water from the front down the perineum to wash the residual bacteria off the skin. Then pat dry with a flannel or kitchen roll just for now. The use of kitchen roll is only for very temporary situations; *never* use loo paper or tissues to dry the perineum after washing, since small pieces of tissue break off and get left to gather bacteria on the skin. Obviously loo paper is fine after passing a stool or if used briefly for dabbing dry after passing urine.

When You Have the Urine Sample Results

Once the results are back, you have more evidence with which to pursue further detective work. The next chapter has more details about this.

Supposing it is positive yet again? Not to worry: your troubles are over because following the advice in this book will stop further attacks. If the result shows a heavy growth *and* the condition is still unstable (that is, you are still feeling lots of twinges), then appropriately sensitive antibiotics should be taken. Three to five days should be enough. Continued sensible drinking, painkillers and urinary voiding will give you comfort and keep decreasing the bacterial growth. Don't overdo the self-help now, just keep comfortable.

Conventional Medical Help

The chances are that you have picked up this book because you haven't got anywhere with the medical profession's help, so it will cheer you up to know that a report from the Institute of Urology states that patient hygiene came out top in a survey of what stops cystitis attacks in young women.

If you haven't tried self-help you will have been subjected to medical 'help'. This currently comprises:

* *Urine samples*
  Mid-stream Urine (MSU)
* *Antibiotics*
  Prescribed whether the MSU is positive or negative
* *Intra-Venous Pyelogram – IVP*
  An X-ray of the kidneys and bladder
* *Cystoscopy*
  The surgeon looks up a cystoscope into the bladder
* *Dilatation*
  Widening or enlarging the urethra or bladder
* *Cauterization*
  Burning away infected and scarred urethral or bladder skin
* *Urodynamics*
  Checking the working of the urinary system
* *Micturating cystogram*
  Measuring the urinary flow

There is a variety of operations to suit particular results of investigations, such as 'bladder washouts', or surgery to correct a prolapsed bladder or to remove stones or obstructions. One good IVP should show whether further urological work is necessary. Do not submit to the surgeon at all if your bladder has behaved perfectly normally until a given incident or time. Look into the particular causes of your infection and try self-help treatments before 'going medical'.

Who Gets Cystitis?

What sort of women get bacterial cystitis? All sorts! Research shows the largest group to be aged 18 to 35 years, but little girls and older women also get it for various reasons. Women who are pregnant form quite a well-known group of bacterial sufferers, and labour can set off a urinary infection. Infections frequently begin during a stay in hospital. In fact, over 30 per cent of all infections contracted in hospital are urinary infections.

Some women never get it, and I am often asked my thoughts on this. There are certain factors that can determine whether a woman will be predisposed to this type of infection:

1. The nearness of the anal opening to the urethral tube varies from woman to woman. Some women may have a good lengthy gap, while others may have a smaller gap. The smaller the gap, the less far germs have to travel.
2. Some women still wipe 'back to front' when they go to the lavatory, enabling germs to enter the urethra easily.
3. Some women may not have a strong enough resistance to the bacteria.
4. Daughters often 'copy' parental hygiene procedures, rightly or wrongly.
5. Failing to pass urine regularly allows germs a longer time to penetrate the urethra and set up a small colony.
6. Some women automatically wash before sex, helping to ensure that germs do not spread from their anal passage to their vagina.
7. Some women shower or bathe after a bowel movement as part of their automatic daily routine.
8. Constipation plays its part, too. There is a big bacterial build-up in large, unpassed faeces. When they are eventually passed there may be a stronger bacterial presence on the anal opening. Many women are frequently constipated, especially before a period.

Chapter 3
GET SOME ANSWERS!

You have never asked for the result of a urine sample? Shame on you. It is *your* sample, not the doctor's. Not only do you have a right to ask what is in it, you absolutely *must*. It is the biggest clue to enable you to start work on the cause or causes of your cystitis.

A positive MSU (mid-stream urine) sample means that infection is present. It will say:

Heavy Growth
Medium Growth
Insignificant Growth
No Growth

The layout of laboratory forms can vary and appear technical. When counselling women, I take account of the following as well as the words:

- any ++ signs against red, white or epithelial cell reports
- whether the woman drank water before taking the sample, which would dilute it
- Whether the patient is under old antibiotic influence

- any reported lessening of symptoms if sympathy antibiotics have been taken during previous attacks. Antibiotics *only* work against infection, nothing else

False results often occur if these factors influenced the sample. I used to think it a good idea to take a 'clearance MSU' after a course of antibiotics. Of course, this would be negative because antibiotics continue their influence for several weeks against a particular bacterium. But other bacteria from the bowel may commence a new bladder infection if not prevented. Therefore I now disagree with taking clearance MSUs, because they can be misleading.

The laboratory will also tell the doctor to which antibiotic group the bacterium is sensitive. A rational choice can then be made, taking into account a variety of factors including the age of the patient, whether she is pregnant or not, etc. If the result says 'mixed growth', domination of the infection by stronger bacteria within it may occur. The first antibiotic may need to be replaced by one sensitive to the dominant bacteria. Only three days need to pass to establish that antibiotics need replacing.

Three full days of any antibiotic is sufficient to tell you whether it has defeated the bacteria. If twingeing rises on the second, third or fourth day, ring the doctor and ask whether the sensitivity culture shows other bacteria or whether there are further antibiotic choices for this bacteria.

You must know the correct sequence of events at this time:

1. Collect the sample under proper conditions.
2. Make sure it arrives in the laboratory during working hours.
3. Make sure there is a full bacterial AND sensitivity culture.
4. Do the three hour management process AFTER the sample has been taken.
5. If it is certainly an infection (i.e. you had neglected hygiene rules) take prescribed antibiotics.

6. If these fail after three days, ring the doctor.
7. Requesting a second urine sample may prove unhelpful since you will have drunk a lot and diluted the bacteria. Also, the first antibiotics may still affect the second sample, giving a false result.
8. It pays to take the first urine sample very seriously.

By the time you get the result, you will have had three days of monitoring your own condition which will help you to decide whether or not to take the recommended drug. Generally, I think that any feeling of discomfort, soreness or twingeing, or swollen and red perineum at this time, should be dealt with by a short course of antibiotics. If vaginal thrush has presented itself on earlier occasions when taking a course of antibiotics, then your doctor should prescribe a 10-day course of Nystatin (known in the US and Australia as Mycostatin) oral tablets together with the best vaginal pessaries. Sporanox or Diflucan (anti-fungal oral treatments) will help just as well.

Just using vaginal pessaries does nothing to treat the intestinal candida upsurge and so, even after completing the pessary course, vaginal thrush may return. Oral tablets help prevent this.

Women who cannot tolerate antibiotics should benefit greatly by the first-aid methods advocated in Chapter 1; daily prevention is important for all women but even more so for them.

Special Clinics

If you do have a sore, swollen or reddened perineum (lie on the bed with a mirror and look!), ring up a special clinic/or genito urinary/medicine outpatients clinic in your nearest large hospital. Say that you think you have a discharge and ask whether you can come in for an examination as soon as possible. These clinics can be walk-ins or by appointment – you will be told which when you telephone. A doctor's referral letter is not required, nor does the clinic's report get sent back to your own doctor.

When you are seen you may be asked whether you have any 'waterworks' trouble as well. Why they can't just say 'urinary symptoms' I can't imagine! 'Waterworks' means sewage and water supply to me!

They will take a urine sample, a vaginal and cervical swab – quite simple, they use a long cotton wool bud – and not only do samples get looked at immediately, but a full three-day culture in the laboratory is also done. A cervical smear is not the same as a cervical swab. The smear tests only for cancer, the swab tests for bacteria. If something is found when they put the specimen under the microscope, you will go home with appropriate treatment according to the condition diagnosed.

Should you be told that there is no infection in the urine or on the swabs in the special clinic, this does not mean that you are 'imagining' your symptoms. It can mean that what is present is not a recognizable sexually transmitted disease. Some of these clinics stick very strictly to reporting only on venereal or sexually transmitted diseases. They do not seem inclined to bend the rules in order to be efficient. It makes no monetary sense to take this attitude and compel the poor patient to use the resources of another department as well. She would have to revisit her doctor, get a referral and wait for an appointment in the gynaecology or urology unit. Then more swabs and microscopes, all costing the clinic money.

Not all special clinics take this strict attitude, and because most women seem, even these days, to have to pluck up some courage to visit one, the doctors mostly do their best to re-assure and to examine gently. Such clinics provide an excellent service – and a free one, if you live in the UK and go to an NHS (National Health Service) clinic. I have used them myself. It is all very good value and you will be seen very quickly.

Another good reason to use the special clinic is to double-check the results reported by the hospital laboratory to which your doctor sent your sample. There are many reasons why your original sample may result in an *in*accurate diagnosis:

- You may have forgotten to refrigerate it at home.
- Once at the doctor's surgery (office) it may again not be refrigerated.
- The collection van may be early, late or not come at all that day, which leaves your sample hanging around.
- It may be a Friday without a late van delivery to the laboratory, so that your sample is not seen until after the weekend!
- You yourself may have taken an unclean specimen.
- Drinking *before* taking the sample dilutes the numbers of bacteria.
- Antibiotics taken near the time the sample was taken always make it negative even if the bacteria are resistant to this antibiotic.

Any or all of these factors could give an *in*accurate result. Only on your local laboratory's past record can you be reasonably certain of how efficient it is – for instance, if *all* your past vaginal swabs have shown positive something or other, or if all your past urine samples have shown positive bacterial counts. By the same token, if they have all shown negative results – in either instance you should use the resources of the special clinic to do a double-check. Or you might want to go to a private specialist to get a second opinion. Ask where the samples are sent, though: if it is the *same* laboratory then you may be wasting your money.

A Positive Sample

So, the urine sample is positive. It is not enough just to know that much. You must ask what the bacterium is called and where it comes from. Most urinary infections are caused by:

- **Escherichia coli** or
- **Streptococcus faecalis**

  then, less commonly, by

- Staphylococcus
- Klebsiella
- Proteus
- Pseudomonas

Pseudomonas is not normal bowel flora – it overgrows like candida if you are given antibiotics. (There is more about all these bacteria in the next chapter.)

These organisms cohabit in the intestines and bowel of every human being. *This means that the infection in your urine sample is due to your own bacteria, which has come from* your *body, no one else's!* This is the most important factor to know when trying to sort yourself out. No doctor *ever* explains this. In short, you are causing your own urinary infection! Ninety-nine per cent of you, all reading this book because you are suffering from urinary infections, are causing your own misery! (Once again I must stress that this applies to women with a proven, named infection in their urine specimens. There are countless other reasons for negative urine samples where the symptoms of cystitis appear the same but the cause or causes have nothing to do with real bacterial infection).

The Truth about Toilet Seats

So, 99 per cent of you are causing your own misery – what about the other 1 per cent? Well, this estimate allows for isolated, unusual infections or even a nasty dose of someone else's bowel bacteria from a badly contaminated lavatory seat. This is very rare, primarily because most women hate unknown lavatories and will either not sit down or will line the seat with tissue paper or lavatory paper. (By the way, never hover! It stops the bladder emptying completely because you are too tense.) If you need to pass a stool in a place other than home, line the seat with toilet roll paper before you sit down. It is the front part of the seat which is potentially the most bacterially contaminated, but it does depend on the place, whether children or old people use it and how often it is cleaned. Perhaps the back part of the seat and the bowl itself look as though they need a good clean? If so, clean the seat and put paper at the back of the seat as well. Bacteria can pass through soft paper and then transfer practically anywhere, which is why cleaning the toilet and washing your hands afterwards are so important.

Passing urine in a strange toilet isn't that tricky. I find that a couple of sheets of paper placed slightly to right of centre allow me to sit on my right side, relaxed enough to empty the bladder fully. The difficulty really comes when there is no paper! Then what? Try one handbag tissue instead. Men don't know how lucky they are!

Always wash your hands afterwards. I do wish that elbow-operated taps and soap dispensers were available in public lavatories, as they are in operating theatres for the surgeons. I hate touching all those taps and soaps and drying facilities with my hands or fingertips; I never really feel clean until I am in my own hotel room or my bathroom at home.

If you are out and in charge of a little girl who wants to go the toilet, you must line the front of the seat and help support her while she goes. When my daughter first began using the loo, I always squatted in front of her and held her under her armpits and around her ribcage. It is so important for such tiny bladders to empty completely and expel any germs around the vulval area. Little girls do tend to want to 'hold it'! They should be told not to, and taught clearly from early years of the dangers of retaining 'nasty germs inside that may start to hurt you'.

If she wants to pass a stool, stay with her and teach her time and again until you are sure she knows no other way than to wipe around her back passage *from behind*. Wiping the back passage from behind and not touching the front is an enormous aid to preventing urinary infection in little girls.

Teach also about lining the seat when they use a toilet away from home, so that a dirty school lavatory doesn't psychologically prevent them from going when they need to.

As a little girl sits on the seat, even if it is lined, she will still want to use her hands on the sides to help support herself. This is unavoidable. Before sitting, she should be taught to break off and hold two or three sheets of paper with which, later, to dab her vulval area dry and then, of course, to wash her hands properly at the basin after pulling the flush.

She should also be shown to put in the basin plug so that hot and cold water can mix to a comfortable temperature for washing her hands. Plenty of soap and rinsing well are good habits to adopt.

Some of you may think this is all very obvious, but would be surprised at how many mothers do not take the time and trouble to get these simple messages across to their daughters. Some years ago, the mother of a five-year-old girl contacted me. Her daughter had constant, proven urinary infections and lived on antibiotics, though scans and examinations all proved negative. When I questioned her, she told me she was only bathing this child once a week! I was patient and practical. The child must be bathed daily. Recently I had cause to ring her, only to find that the now eight-year-old girl is frequently hospitalized, her life painful and still disrupted with infections.

'You are bathing her daily as I said?'

'Well, not really, we're busy and I forget, I suppose it's my fault really, she baths every three or four days.'

I was almost speechless with rage and told her so in great fury. Why hadn't the doctors asked about hygiene habits and, upon being told, refused to treat her daughter until the daily bath was in place? This constitutes neglect, I think, on the mother's part.

I can't bear not to say a word about small boys here! It is not so much for their sake that I do as for the sake of their future girlfriends and wives. I took just as much trouble over my son's lavatorial behaviour and habits as my daughter's. This extends even to basin tidiness and to cleaning round the bath for the next person.

At aged eight my son was taught to clean a lavatory correctly and I still make him practise it during the holidays – and he's 20 now! If my children leave any kind of unacceptable mess in my bathroom, they get told instantly to come and wipe round. I just will not let them get away with it.

Many is the time that I have been asked shyly during a counselling session the best way to clean a lavatory. It is hard to believe that young women often don't know, but it is true. Older women are, of course, more learned and practised. So here, for you younger ones, is the method that works best:

1. Keep cream cleaner and a heavy string cloth in a bowl or on a peg (I've got an antique chamber pot for mine!) in the bathroom. Also a good brush-cleaning set.
2. Lift the seat and squirt some cream cleaner around the bowl. Scrub the bowl all round with the long-handled toilet brush.
3. Flush and scrub again, finally rinsing the brush under the last fresh water flowing into the bowl.

4. Now wet the string cloth under the hot tap and squirt a few drops of cream cleaner onto it.
5. Clean the topside of the lavatory seat first, then the underside and lastly the rim of the porcelain bowl.
6. Thoroughly rinse the cloth in hot water.
7. Now wipe the cream cleaner off the porcelain rim, then off the underside of the seat. Rinse the cloth again.
8. Repeat item 7 and then wipe the cream cleaner off the topside of the seat.
9. Rinse the open cloth (don't scrunch it into a ball) thoroughly under hot running water.
10. Now wipe that topside of the seat once more.
11. Rinse the cloth well for a final time, squeeze it and leave it hanging exposed to air and well ventilated over the edge of the bowl in which it is kept.

You notice that I haven't mentioned disinfectants at all. I don't believe they are necessary in the first place and, in the second, disinfectant on the lavatory seat itself can cause horrible skin troubles (it is not a problem in the pan unless 'splashback' happens when a stool is passed). I have specifically mentioned using a cream cleaner because you can see traces of it if you haven't thoroughly wiped it off. It is this kind of cleaner that I use at home and I find it meets my own (very stringent!) standards.

Trichomonas

Trichomonas is worth mentioning here. It causes a nasty vaginal discharge and you can get a vicious dose of cystitis or urethritis from it. Trichomonas is a water-borne parasite which lives in lavatory pan water. If your lavatory pan is quite deep and the water splashes back onto your bottom when you pass a stool, the trichomonal parasite can splash onto your skin. Wiping it with loo paper won't work. The parasite quickly swims in the vulval moisture and starts to breed in vaginal moisture. Once there it can also be transmitted by sexual intercourse.

Trichomonas dies in air and lives in moisture. What stops the 'splash-back' is to place a sheet of paper on the surface of the water in the pan. This effectively prevents water from leaving the pan.

The more people using a lavatory, the more it needs cleaning. Flat- or house-shares involving several young people require a lot of lavatory cleaning. If you have been getting urinary infections regularly, keep the cream cleaner and cloth in your own room and clean that lavatory *before* you personally use it. When it is clean, just dab the seat dry with some loo paper before you sit on it, so that you can happily discount the seat as the remotest source of infection and so that you can do the essential bottle-washing (described in Chapter 5).

What Happens to Your Urine Sample?

Returning to swabs and urine samples, the one and only request that I make prior to a counselling appointment is – 'please ring your doctor and ask for photocopies of the results of swabs and MSUs to bring with you.' I used to be satisfied with verbal reports, but no longer.

It is absolutely extraordinary that so many victims of urinary infection don't know what is in their urine sample results.

When you take your sample it needs to be collected carefully, as I have said. If you and your doctor are working well together you should be allowed two or three spare sterile sample jars with labels so that you can take a specimen early, if a new attack starts.

When your clean urine sample arrives at a hospital laboratory, having been personally delivered or taken by the collecting van which picks them up from the doctor, it is checked in, much like a guest arriving at a hotel reception!

Although out-patients' urine samples do not arrive till mid-morning, the laboratory is already at work, if it is within a large hospital, checking in samples from the various wards. A steady number of hospital porters and orderlies comes to the reception desk with bundles of samples of all sorts from all over the hospital and the local health authority catchment area. Some days can be busy – for instance on days when local ante-natal clinics are held and routine samples sent off to the hospital laboratory.

The laboratory usually works six days a week, but emergency work will be done on a Sunday! In the laboratory where I followed the processing of urine samples, they have their own in-house procedures or protocol. All hospitals are free to make their own protocol, but every laboratory in the UK is subjected to regular spot-checks by a special central public health laboratory.

At the reception desk, two sorters separate sample jars, which should be (but are not always) clearly labelled, from their forms upon which the doctor has stated a request for analysis together with the patient's details.

The details from the doctor are *instantly*, right there at the reception desk, computerized and the specimen given a number on the screen. The computer details are then printed out onto a sticker which is stuck on the back of the original form. All these forms are taken through to the offices of the various microbiologists, who then decide which samples should be looked at under a microscope in addition to the culturing overnight which *all* samples undergo.

All urine samples – from urological hospitals especially, or from the urological ward within the general hospital – are automatically sent for microscopy (put under the microscope) as well as culture. Any others are judged by sight if they are cloudy with pus and blood or clear, and then added on to the others indicated for microscopy. For some specific clinical indications it is useful to look for pus cells or peculiar red cells. The microbiologist is very dependent on having the form filled in properly.

Computer No.	*001*
Patient's No.	*45*
Patient's name, birth date, sex	*Bloggs, 28/11/41, Female*
Consultant's Name	*Mr Waterflow*
Location	*General Hospital, Looe*
Doctor	*L. Bowl, MD*
Specimen No.	*287 (written on lid of jar)*
Investigation type	*MSU culture and sensitivity*
Antibiotics	*None taken recently*
Diagnosis?	*Urinary infection*

The computer has an individual number for each patient and for each specimen, which is distinct from the specimen's new number freshly inked on the lid of the specimen jar.

While the forms are with the microbiologists in their offices, the actual urine specimens mount up quickly enough into a tray-load. This tray is carried down a long room to the 'urine bench'. Other benches are for other specimens – respiratory, gynaecological, wounds, faecal, leukaemic and neonatal, for example. HIV (AIDS) patients' specimens have their own bench in a separate room.

On the urine bench the tray-load is placed onto a 'cold table' which is refrigerated to keep the specimens in a good state until they are ready to be 'plated', i.e. when small amounts of urine are put onto a special culture dish or plate.

A medical laboratory scientific officer – MLSO for short – is now in charge of the specimens. He or she may set up as few as 250 specimens a day on culture plates or far more than that. Double-checking specimen number against culture plate number is of prime importance. Let's follow Rita Bloggs' specimen:

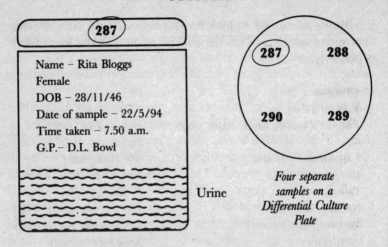

Name – Rita Bloggs
Female
DOB – 28/11/46
Date of sample – 22/5/94
Time taken – 7.50 a.m.
G.P.– D.L. Bowl

Urine

Four separate samples on a Differential Culture Plate

Figure 3: Urine sample form; four separate samples on a differential quarter culture plate

The MLSO writes up a batch of numbers on the differential culture plates – four numbers per plate. Differential culture (also called culture quarter) plates are thin, clear round plastic holders with tops. The numbers go clockwise in quarters and mistakes are seldom made.

The MLSO then prepares to put a droplet of Rita's urine into the quarter of the plate containing her number. The plate has a green/agar/protein film (green = dye; agar = seaweed protein; other proteins and carbohydrates = bacterial food source) upon which most of the possible organisms in Rita's urine will grow. The shaken urine jar is placed on a green paper towel so that any spillage gets absorbed. In sterile packaging on the bench are thin *bacterial loops*. Each loop is a long, fine plastic stick which, when the end is dipped in the urine, retains just one precise microlitre. This microlitre of urine (droplet) is smeared onto Rita's section of the quarter culture plate.

The object of the culture is to give a rough idea of how many organisms are grown on the plate overnight. Several other methods may be used, but laboratories usually end up doing the simplest thing because there are so many specimens to process.

A positive MSU is taken as one where there are more than 10,000 organisms of a single type present in one millilitre of urine. If the MSU was not taken cleanly by the patient, or if the specimen has hung around for a while, there may be more than one organism present. This is a mixed growth of doubtful significance. Your doctor may have to order another MSU. If there are strong second and third organisms present, the MSU may have been contaminated from extra outside factors and an unclean sample, again necessitating another MSU. Less than 10,000 organisms per millilitre are present in normal urine from people without symptoms, and would be recorded as an absence of infection. Do follow my previous instructions for collecting a clean MSU, because you will help the laboratory to give an accurate result first time and save the NHS a lot of time and money.

After plating the urine samples, the smeared plates are stacked on top of each other upside down so that any condensation forming on the inside of the lid does not drop into the growing bacteria. At the end of the day all the plates are racked and taken to the Hot Room. Here, at 37°C/98.6°F (body temperature), the organisms have all night to reproduce.

The remaining urine in each sample jar is refrigerated for two more days, in case more is required for a different test. If not, then after two days the jars are autoclaved (whizzed round) until sterile; the urine, now clear of organisms, is thrown down the plug-hole; and the empty jars are sent off to be incinerated.

In the mean time, the microbiologists have decided from the doctors' forms which additional samples should also have microscopy (examination under a microscope.)

The MLSO then collects those sample jars chosen by the microbiologists for microscopy. Wearing protective gloves, he or she shakes up the contents of each jar again, then dips the discardable end of a fixed-volume (60-microlitre) Finn pipette into Rita's urine specimen jar. The pipette sucks up exactly 60 microlitres of her urine, then releases it into a small hole in a flat-bottomed tray.

The MLSO then uses an *inverted* microscope to look at the urine from *underneath* so that the organisms can be clearly seen. The MLSO is looking for pus cells, red cells, squamous cells, casts and crystals.

Pus cells	Indicate inflammation
Red cells	Indicate blood contamination
Squamous cells	Are broken off skin cells from, say, the urethral or vaginal lining – indicating contamination
Casts from kidney tissues	Indicate disease of the kidneys
Crystals	Occur in certain urological conditions

Whatever the MLSO sees, it is only a visual, the real 'meaty' results of Rita's MSU will be what has grown overnight on the culture plate.

What is seen under the inverted microscope is entered on a very small label to be stuck on the original doctor's form.

Pus cells are counted; if above 10 cells show, it is a probable UTI (urinary tract infection).

If Red and Squamous cells are seen, then 10 cells = Few; under 100 cells = Moderate, over 100 cells = Numerous, indicating the likelihood of infection.

All the doctors' forms, now with a lot of information gathering on them, are put in order of urine specimen number to await the addition of the next day's plate culture growth report.

At about 9 a.m. the next morning, the MLSO begins examining the differential culture plates, writing in brief on the back of the form what has been found. Each plate and its four cultures are made clearly visible under a strong light. The MLSO is trained to spot the obvious bacterial groups and then to implement further instant tests and more overnight tests if the precise organism growth has not yet revealed itself.

In the laboratory, approximately 70 per cent of all positive urine samples show a Coliform growth. Next come *Staphylococcus, Streptococcus, Pseudomomas, Proteus and Klebsiella,* making up between them the other 30 per cent. All are bacteria from our *own* bowels.

A lot of mixed infections come up and, despite the obvious differences to the naked eye of sparse, medium or heavy plate organism growth, the laboratory protocol (procedure) dictates that no further testing is done and the result then given as it stands to the requesting doctor. The understanding is that the doctor will tell the patient to take another sample, as the mixed infection is felt to be indicative of an unclean specimen. The patient should be taught to take a fresh clean early-morning specimen and to get it to the lab quickly.

Antibiotics have probably already been prescribed and taken, even before the sample result has come through. This is bad luck but should not alter the enthusiasm with which specimens are taken early on in infections.

In addition to a tremendous range of bacteria-proving tests, the microbiology laboratory also has to recommend to the patient's doctor an antibiotic to which the bacteria are sensitive:

'*sensitive to*' means bacteria *cannot* grow or thrive

'*resistant to*' means bacteria *can* still grow and thrive

So another culture plate is set up on night two or three of the urine sample's stay in the laboratory. This next plate is called a Sensitivity plate; there is room for only six small discs on each plastic Lysed Blood Agar Sensitivity plate. With a laboratory loop the MLSO scrapes up a tiny amount of the

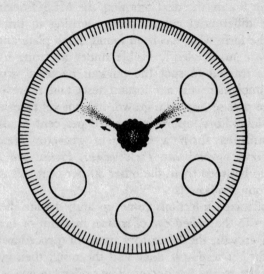

Figure 4: Lysed Blood Agar Sensitivity plate

organisms grown on the differential plates overnight and sets it gently down in the centre of the Sensitivity plate. The edge of the plate is spread with a 'control' fully-sensitive organism. Each disc is impregnated with a different antibiotic and set near the outer edge of the plate. Overnight the organisms grow where they can on the plate. They will grow around 'friendly' antibiotics but appear to stay away from 'unfriendly' ones. Hence they are 'resistant to' or 'sensitive to' an antibiotic.

These again get a night in the Hot Room at 37°C/98.6°F.

There are four main sets/groups of antibiotics tested on the Sensitivity plate. Each of the four sets contains up to six antibiotics which are especially good for fighting urinary infections. Most organisms are sensitive to all of these. Second-degree and third-degree sets are used for resistant coliforms and pseudomonas; fourth degree sets for staphlyococci.

Set 1
Ampicillin/Amoxycillin
Sulphamethoxazole
Trimethoprim
Nalidixic Acid
Nitrofurantoin
Caphadroxil

Set 2
Ampicillin/Amoxycillin
Augmentin
Gentamicin

Ciproflaoxacin
Cefuroxime

Teicoplanin

Set 3
Azlocillin
Azlocillin
Netilmicin
Amikacin
Ceftazidime

Set 4
Azlocillin
Penicillin
Methicillin
  (Flucloxacillin)
Novibiocin
Rifampicin
Tetracycline

Fusidic Acid

Other sets of less well-known antibiotics can be tested when required, or the MLSO can arrange for just one special antibiotic to be tested by itself.

It is while these professionals are at work on her sample that Rita should use the first-aid management process to keep herself as comfortable as possible. Once their report is through, further help, possibly with antibiotics or by using the methods outlined in later chapters of this book, can commence.

Once the full range of tests is accomplished, your doctor is sent the report, the laboratory computer updated with the final diagnosis and the old culture plates autoclaved and incinerated.

Now What?

So you've got your result! *You've asked for it* from your doctor and now *you know* whether it is a case of pure named infection or not. The next piece of the puzzle is to know where the bacteria come from.

Chapter 4

WHERE DO THE BACTERIA COME FROM?

The vast majority of bacteria in a urinary infection come from the body's intestines and bowels – 'the intestinal tract' as doctors call it.

How Do Bacteria Get into the Intestines?

All the bacterial micro-organisms found in the gut are present in the air, on the ground and in all water. They enter the food chain at many points. They could be resting on a plate of food, or introduced by contaminated hands during food preparation, or through liquid intake. When the weather is humid and moist, they breed in greater numbers and we even breathe them in! We obviously also eat them as a matter of daily habit, but we first acquire them at birth or very shortly afterwards from the air, the birth environment and our mother's milk. Micro-organisms enter into our intestines and stay there for the rest of our days! They are in fact what is known as 'the normal flora', an essential part of our resistance to infection.

The amounts and kinds of bacteria present in our system

change continually. Old bacteria die and new ones reproduce. The balance of them all in relation to one another is what keeps them all occupied. If one lot overgrows, the others attack – if they don't, the body may succumb to an overwhelming bacterial infection; left untreated by antibiotics this would lead to the death of the person and the death of the other bacterial colonies. So they fight within us for their own survival. We remain totally unaware of all this activity, thank goodness!

While thus kept busily occupied with their own life and death, the many groups of enterobacteria (those specifically living in the intestines) cause us no trouble at all. They may even be helpful in breaking down particles of enzymes, proteins, fats and acids which are left at the end of the digestion of food. But trouble does arise if they overgrow, such as if we eat large amounts of carbohydrates (enterobacteria love to eat carbohydrate particles), or if they get outside the intestinal tract where there are fewer colonies of enemy bacteria to fight them off.

A person's immune-system response is therefore important, so the very young, very old, sick or dying can become terribly ill with enterobacterial overgrowths. Particularly common sites of infections are the lungs and the urinary tract – hence urinary infection. The infection to the lungs travels either in the bloodstream or through ordinary breathing. Infection of the urinary tract occurs when external perineal bacteria, which have come out of the bowels, travel up and into the urethral tube and bladder.

The Discovery of Bacteria

How on earth has all this unseen life within us been discovered? It cannot be seen with the naked eye, so could the doctors be making it all up?

Until just over a 120 years ago, micro-organisms could not

be discovered because the compound microscope had not been invented. Only simple glass lenses with insufficient powers of magnification existed. These simple lenses were first used in the 13th century and no improvements were made to them for another 250 years. Then in the 1650s a Dutchman, Antony Van Leewenhoek, made his own simple lenses to try to satisfy his curiosity about living things like plants, water and scrapings from bad teeth, blood or animal manure.

He had no laboratory, though, and there was no knowledge of culture growth. He couldn't grow organisms, only look at patterns of colours on seemingly lifeless objects. Nevertheless, he could just about make out some of those organisms that did not die straight away when put under his lenses. He drew them and reported what he could about them but it was still a pretty hopeless state of affairs. Not until the 19th century – with Louis Pasteur, Koch, Weigert, Salomonsen and Hoffman and brilliant additional discoveries from Ehrlich, Loeffler, Ziel and Nielson – were microscopes upgraded and improved. The techniques of growing cultures and of staining slides with colours to show up colourless bacteria then enabled the modern science of microbiology to really take off.

The culture plates described in the previous chapter were first invented by Oscar Brefeld in 1872, who was later helped by Frau Hesse and a Mr Petri, who came up with the final version in 1882 of what is still used in laboratories today for the growing/cultivating of bacteria. They are even known as Petri plates (or dishes)!

Thus it is only within the last 120 years that scientists have discovered the world of unseen bacteria. For each species and sub-species scientists have invented names and numbers for identifying and referencing them. And the discovery continues: recently, while visiting a laboratory, a technician found a bacterium he had never seen before. Can you imagine the excitement! Like holding a new baby, I should think!

The Bacteria of the Intestines

We know that faeces carry solid waste material out of our bodies; we are not going to investigate it all here. What we are interested in are the six main groups of aerobic (oxygen-loving) bacteria that cause infections of the urine, urethra and bladder. These can mount higher up the system into the kidneys and then into the bloodstream so that you may feel dreadfully unwell all over.

A normal, bacterially balanced, easily passed stool doesn't smell nasty, but if you are ill with some kind of infection or virus it may be quite offensive. During the acute phase of mercury poisoning from my amalgams and added gold caps, both stools and urine literally sank. I know now that this was because of methyl mercury being formed during metal corrosion. If stools and urine are always offensive this is abnormal.

The groups of bacteria are members of a 'super-group' called *Enterobacteriaceae*, which includes:

Escherichia
Klebsiella
Proteus
(which are part of the *Coliform* group)
Pseudomonas
Staphylococcus
Streptococcus
(which are part of the *Coccus* group)

but over 100 other types of organisms are quite normally found in stool analyses. There are a hundred times as many *anaerobes* – organisms which prefer to grow in the absence of oxygen – than aerobes, but strangely they do not commonly cause urinary infection.

Coliforms

Coliforms sub-divide into many numbered individual kinds. The commonest is *Escherichia coli*, and within that group the O-numbers of 1, 2, 6, 7, 11, 15 and 75 cause more urinary infections than others. Why the name 'Escherichia'? In 1866 a man in Germany called Herr Escherich discovered these rod-shaped bacteria in the faeces of babies. Although he called them *Bacillus*, we now know them as coliforms and the commonest variety as Escherichia coli.

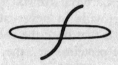

Figure 5: A coliform

The rod-shaped coliforms are, of course, only microscopic in size. They are measured in microns (one micron is a thousandth of a millimetre). Coliforms are measured at about 1 unit wide and 5–8 units long. They swim in moisture and multiply extremely quickly, dividing every 20 minutes under best conditions. After 24 hours on the differential plate in the Hot Room at 37°C/98.6°F, the culture plate is covered in coliforms, as easily obvious to the naked eye as the letters on this page.

Most coliforms are very mobile because of their *flagellae*, which act as oars running the width of the rod from side to side. As well as needing a moist or wet environment, food – in the form of sugars of all sorts, carbohydrates and proteins, all of which are present from human ingestion in our intestines – is essential to their survival. Coliforms reproduce themselves continuously by dividing and subdividing, the rate dependent upon the conditions in our intestines, i.e. the meals we have eaten in the past 24 hours, or how well our immune system is functioning to keep the colony numbers self-regulatory. If we are ill already, the coliform colonies will overgrow because other bacteria are too busy with the illness to find time to fight the coliforms off.

Our body temperature of 37°C/98.6°F, in which the microbiologists grow laboratory cultures of coliforms, is also normal for the human body. Higher temperatures may produce a higher rate of bacterial reproduction, lower body temperatures may slow down the bacterial activity.

What all this shows is that human beings provide the perfect environment for some bacterial growth. Everything these little bugs want, we can provide in never-ending amounts. One quite interesting point is that once the coliforms are overgrowing, reducing stocks of proteins, etc., they die because of their own overgrowth. I have talked in past years to doctors who have shrugged off urinary infections as 'self-regulating' in that after three or four days the bacteria are dying or dead because they have depleted their own living conditions too much to be able to sustain their own reproduction.

I seem to remember telling these doctors that if they personally had ever had an attack of cystitis they would not want to wait on without treatment or first aid to see if it went away by itself! There is also the matter of the risk of infecting the kidneys.

Proteus

Both Proteus and Klebsiella, of the coliform group, are names often reported on MSU forms. Proteus bacteria are rod-shaped. They are 0.5 units wide but only 1–3 units long. They swarm together on some culture plates and need their own additional laboratory test since they can resemble the Pseudomonas group of bacteria. The flagellae enable them to swim well in moisture and they prefer temperatures between 20 and 40°C/68 and 104°F – they quite enjoy their night in the Hot Room! Like so many other inhabitants of the intestines, they cause no trouble unless they stray from their normal habitat. Once in the bladder they act viciously, repeatedly causing lesions and bleeding from old scars in the lining. They use the urea in the urine and make ammonia, which makes the urine alkaline (opposite of acid). This sometimes leads to 'infection stone' formation. Making the urine alkaline with bicarbonate, Cymalon/Cystopurin or potassium citrate, as mentioned in the first-aid method on pages 15-16, does not therefore inhibit a Proteus infection.

Figure 6: Proteus bacillus

Klebsiella

Klebsiella are bacillus that live by themselves, seldom joining up except occasionally in twos. They are static souls and, to protect themselves from frequent attack by other inhabitants of the intestines, produce a kind of slime that defeats attackers. Although they live by themselves, such is the world of microorganisms that 'singles' colonies form on the culture plates!

They look more oval in shape than either rod or circular and vary from 0.5–1.0 units wide and 1–3 units long.

Figure 7: Klebsiella bacillus

Growth occurs at 37°C/98.6°F; killing them off would require boiling them for 20 minutes of 60°C/140°F. I find all these temperatures and times staggering: for me they beg the question of what temperature a human being would finally die at if boiled!

Cocci

Staphylococcus

Staphylococcus, part of the Coccus group, look quite different from coliforms and are only 1 unit in diameter, being circular in shape. Staphs, as we will call them, tend to cluster together, much like a diamond-cluster engagement ring. There are three main groups of staphs but others do exist.

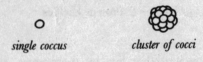

single coccus   *cluster of cocci*

Figure 8: Staphylococcus

Staphs are part of the normal flora found on healthy skin, particularly where there are folds in the skin like those on the perineum. In overgrowth staphs create pus; they are also found in boils, nasal infections and lung infections. Some strains may also lead to infection of the blood vessels in bones and resultant osteomyelitis. Bladder catheters are a source of staph infection. Some types of staph cause UTI (urinary tract infection) more readily than others.

Staphs are one of the main hospital-induced infections, being present in the nasal cavities and colds of hospital staff and patients where warmth and weakened resistance help to make an exceptional environment for staph reproduction. They can also grow, unlike coliforms, in a wider variety of temperatures ranging from 12°C/53.6°F to 45°C/113°F, and produce great colonies in only 18 hours!

They eat the usual particles of proteins, carbohydrates and sugars, which reach the outer skin surface via either a cut on the skin or a boil. The many moist mucous secretions of the nose, throat, lungs, vagina, vulva and perineum are rich in environmental delights of bacterial food and transportation. Funnily enough, if you have a cut and the staph exudes pus, that pus scab acts as a physical barrier to the further spread of staphs – sadly, the same effect doesn't happen in a bladder infection where the urine and lack of air promote, rather than prevent, the staph from spreading because scabs cannot form in wetness.

Staph is so prevalent now, especially in hospitals, that its own geneticism has begun to produce an enzyme that is resistant to most antibiotics. Other than by antibiotics, the bacteria can be killed during sterilization with strong antiseptics or by boiling at 70°C/158°F for 30 minutes.

Streptococcus
Streptococcus look the same as Staphylococcus but form up in chains rather than clusters, which is one of the determining differences assessed under the laboratory microscope.

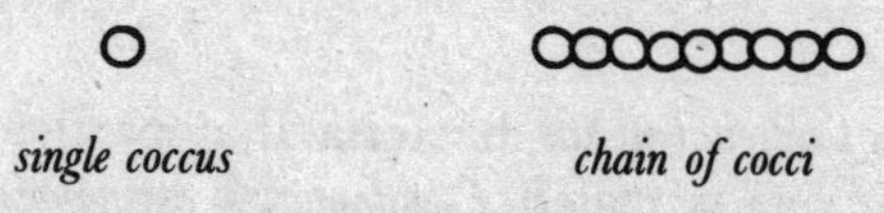

single coccus   chain of cocci

Figure 9: Streptococcus

There are three main groups of Streps but, again, many others exist.

Strep Pyogenes and Strep Pneumoniae Both these groups of Streps live in the nasal cavities and throat. If access to the bloodstream has occurred, antibodies will gather at the site and mostly succeed in repelling the invasion. Not always, though, and *Strep pyogenes* infections are responsible for throat and ear infections, local skin infections (anywhere), scarlet fever and childbirth fever. *Strep pneumoniae* will cause upper respiratory infections such as pneumonia, blood sepsis or meningitis.

Strep Faecalis (or *Enterococcus faecalis*, as it is now known) is a really dire one when it comes to urinary infection since, like coliforms, it lives in the bowels on a permanent basis. Once a stool is passed, *Strep faecalis* stays on the perineum, enabling bacterial penetration of the urethra and bladder, just like coliforms.

Its primary food is sugar but it also draws nutrients from mucous and blood. It, too, can reproduce under low temperatures or high temperatures, making virtually all environments and weather conditions favourable.

Once *streptococci* have invaded the urethra and bladder, growing colonies can cause lesions (cuts or breaks) in the surface skin, encouraging bleeding and the exudation of pus into the urine. With every microscopic or minute lesion (graze), a scar remains to give less resistance to the next bacterial invasion. My own years of recurrent urinary infections in the 1960s and early 1970s saw bleeding start just 40 minutes after the first signalling urethral 'twinge'.

Pseudomonas

The strain of *Pseudomonas* bacteria that particularly carries human infections is called *Pseudomonas aeruginosa* and rarely grows in the intestines, skin or throat. It usually erupts into an infection when there is an existing lesion (graze or cut), or when the intestinal balance is poor. Catheters, urethral operations and antibiotics tend to encourage *Pseudomonas*.

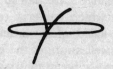

Figure 10: Pseudomonas bacillus

Each rod is thinner than those of a *coliform* and shorter in length, measurements being 0.5 units wide and 1.5–3.0 units long. It can also be called *Pseudomonas pyocyanea* (green pigment) and is a fast mover, having one flagella which branches into three waving 'oars' (see Figure 10). It loves the 37°C/98.6°F of the laboratory Hot Room but can reproduce at 5°C/41°F or anything else up to 45°C/113°F! A higher temperature will kill it off.

Antibiotics

So one or more of these six horrible bacteria have been reported by the microbiology laboratory to your doctor. Remember the laboratory also tested for antibiotic sensitivity? Perhaps some very generalized information on these medications might round off this chapter nicely.

I never knew it, but antibiotics act in two ways: either by effectively preventing bacteria from reproducing (such action being termed 'bacteriostatic') *or* by actually killing them through bactericidal action.

Of the common antibiotics, Penicillin, Streptomycin and Neomycin act bactericidally. Tetracyclines, Sulphonamides and Chloramphenicol act bacteriostatically.

The action of antibiotics on each strain of bacteria varies enormously. Over the years, scientists working for the major pharmaceutical companies have had to discover and document the precise ways in which bacteria react to each drug and exactly how they are killed off or curtailed.

Patients should be well aware of the general action of broad-spectrum treatment, since when the balance of intestinal bacteria is affected, yeast infections can take a big hold in the gut. Secondary infections of the same sort, having not been completely killed, can rapidly overgrow as a reaction to the death of most of their number and the need to get back to full colony strength.

An obvious additional factor to the laboratory's recommended antibiotic is whether you are allergic to it. Any side-effects – such as sickness or diarrhoea occurring in the first hours or days of administration – should be reported to your doctor and the drug's suitability should be reassessed. You should probably not take any of that class of antibiotic again in the future.

There is also no doubt that these gut bacteria are cunning little bugs! They are quite able, over time, to become resistant by changing genetically or by producing an enzyme which might render a newly administered antibiotic incapable of its own ordinary, expected activity. In other words, these bacteria learn to adapt faster than pharmaceutical scientists do!

Chlamydia and Candida

Two other bacteria most women have heard about in relation to urinary problems are worth a mention here. The first is

Chlamydia, which we all know about from vaginal swab tests and magazine articles. *Chlamydia trachomatis* is the strain associated with urethritis and cervicitis.

Chlamydia does not inhabit the intestines like the others, but instead acts like a parasite, invading and then setting up home in the cytoplasm of epithelial 'skin' cells.

It seems that chlamydial infection can be transmitted from one person to another. Transmission is by sexual contact, during which skin cells are passed on and the parasite goes as well. In women, the infection is in the cervix as well as the urethra, so vaginal discharge may be a symptom.

The second extra organism is that well-known fungus called *candida*. I mention it here in defiance of all those doctors who do not seem to accept that candida can be present in the bladder and cause cystitis.

Candida starts out life in exactly the same manner as described for other intestinal inhabitants, but can also be found in all mucous areas of the body. Only when the body becomes severely debilitated, diabetic or immuno-suppressed from antibiotics or disease will the candida fungus overgrow. I have written much about candida in my other books, so here I just want to talk about it in terms of the urethra and bladder.

Indwelling urinary catheters may introduce candida to the bladder; long-term antibiotics and inflammatory lesions of the bladder lining may predispose a woman to bladder Candidosis; candida is carried in the bloodstream (which has an alkaline pH) and the presence of yeast-infected blood in bladder urine may help maintain the alkalinity, thus providing a welcome habitat.

After antibiotics, bladder urine may carry yeast organisms that have overgrown in the intestine and are being passed out via blood filtration in the kidneys. Candida is sometimes cited on death certificates as a contributory factor in severely sick patients. It is capable of travelling to every organ of the body in the blood vessels and needs to be taken more seriously by microbiologists and doctors in relation to the great social and physical suffering which so-called vaginal thrush can cause.

Controlling the Bacteria

The artificial control of bacteria in our bodies for the purposes of understanding urinary infections is expensive in terms of labour, time, equipment, sampling, doctors, paperwork, antibiotics and patients' suffering. If these bacteria are *normally* in our intestines and *normally* cause no trouble except when outside the intestines and doing some perineal travelling, there must be some way, not involving man-made microbiological and pharmaceutical intervention, of preventing that bacterial travel, trouble and expense for the patient. Apart from a debilitating course of antibiotics, what other course of action can you, the patient, take?

Chapter 5

HOW CAN I STOP THE BACTERIA?

Quite simply, you can't 'stop' bacteria – but you *can* control them. Such bacteria have been as much a part of human biology as our arms and legs, since we were primevally formed. Every animal has them, too.

I am going to divide this chapter into two parts. The first is backed by research done in the 1960s by the renowned Royal Navy surgeon Captain Cleave. The second part shows the 100 per cent efficacy of practical hygiene procedures in preventing urinary infections – my own discovery arrived at over years of trial and error.

We Are What We Eat

Surgeon Captain Cleave, now deceased, was a much travelled Royal Navy surgeon with a distinct interest in research. He was sometime Director of Medical Research at the Royal Navy Medical School in Hampshire and spent most of his medical life being fascinated by the health of the naval men under his care. On spells of shore leave abroad he amused himself by collecting data on the dietary habits of many different races of people, most frequently on the Indian and African continents. He would compare these with the diets of his own Western naval patients. In the years after the Second World War he began to witness increasing ill health in the Western world and among his men.

Food Refining

What we eat, which ends up as faeces in our bowels, starts out by entering our mouths. The process of refining the tough fibres from cereals, pulses, fruits and vegetables has very slowly evolved since Anglo-Saxon times, but quickened up from the 19th century when presumably the Industrial Revolution and an easier export/import trade made commercializing food a desirable money-making industry. The addition of refined white sugars to virtually every meal in some way or other, increasing to saturation point in the latter 20th century, is a much discussed topic by the guardians of our health education today.

White flour, sieved and bleached to remove the brown fibrous outer husks, was originally known only to the stomachs of well-to-do Greek farmers and nobility as long ago as 500 BC. By the 1800s virtually everyone everywhere was eating it, in all strata of society.

Hippocrates in his medical school on Kos used white flour specifically as a medicine for arresting diarrhoea, since he noticed how much more slowly it passed through a patient's gut into the faeces. Refined white flour is much stickier when mixed in moisture and stays longer in the intestines. As the starch in the flour ferments into sugar, that sugar spends longer in the intestines – enabling all bacteria normally resident in the intestines to multiply more easily, since they are not constantly kept on the move.

Peristaltic waves are muscular ripples or contractions of the colon walls which push faeces along and into the bowels for evacuation, a bit like the way a snake moves.

If the peristaltic waves are slowed, constipation results. Bacterial multiplication is then far greater. Human genetic machinery cannot cope with the bacterial build-up, so the maintenance of a good, healthy digestive system becomes extremely difficult.

When sugar refining began from sugar cane and sugar beet it was too laborious to provide for general consumption and so again, only the rich had access to it. In fact, it wasn't exported to Britain until the 12th century, but from the end of the 18th century consumption rates rocketed, reaching all areas of society.

Thus the 'sweet tooth' is a multi-million pound industry the world over – drinks and sweets manufacturers being two of the major monetary beneficiaries.

Apart from the rise in the incidence of tooth decay that accompanies the increased consumption of white flour and white sugar, all sorts of illnesses connected with the digestive process have increased in prevalence, including ulcers, irritable bowel syndrome, diverticulitis, varicose veins, haemorrhoids, obesity, candida, diabetes and urinary infections. Surgeon Captain Cleave produced large numbers of charts and diagrams to support all this, and indeed I think we could all admit to knowing that refined foods are less good for us, even if we don't technically know why.

Basically, our digestive tracts teem with vicious bacteria whose levels depend largely on how long the food process takes in the intestines. The quicker that food is passed through and out of the bowels, the fewer bacteria thrive. If your system is slow, you will allow greater numbers of bacteria to multiply.

Husks on oats and wheat are the fibre which helps maintain a faster, more regular bowel evacuation. Nevertheless, many people are allergic to cereal. Individual experiment is the way to encourage a faster digestion and evacuation. Surgeon

Captain Cleave always recommended starting with small amounts of bran (a teaspoonful), if at all, and building up to a level that ensures a comfortable daily bowel movement. He felt that changing from white flour to whole meal flour and the avoidance of all white sugar should be sufficient in itself to get a daily bowel movement, but he recognized that this was dependent upon each person's metabolic rate. There is no doubt in my mind that sugar in all forms and from all sources causes constipation. Cut it out and stools become looser and regular.

With regular bowel movements, bacterial build-up and toxic products are kept at low levels. These bacteria and products primarily include all the natural bacteria that are, as a rule, in the intestines to aid digestion. When they overgrow, they run riot. Surgeon Captain Cleave also stresses strongly not to overeat. The bacterial response to large amounts of food is to multiply faster because the food requires larger bacterial colonies to help break it down – naturally, they multiply to deal with this extra workload.

Reducing the Levels of Coliforms
in the Intestines

Three rules exist to help maintain smaller levels of coliforms in the gut:

1. Don't overeat (as this encourages coliform growth).
2. Don't eat white flour or sugar (as this feeds the coliform bacteria).
3. Don't get constipated (as this retains old bacteria).

Eating bran rather than cutting out sugar may even cause more constipation. If you only take wheat bran, the ridged colon may clog up with the fine wheat particles. The particles become impacted and actually begin to create constipation instead of stopping it. Eating oat bran as well is better: the oat bran in porridge, which is larger, prevents the finer wheat bran from this sedimentary build-up, and allows each its own uniquely helpful action if used occasionally. Too many eggs can also be a prime cause of constipation; two or three a week are acceptable.

So that's how to reduce coliform levels from within – but what about tackling them from without?

Conventional Medicine

For years the medical profession has been besieged by growing numbers of women patients with urinary tract infection (UTI), yet medical schools have failed to address this problem. Lectures on UTI are usually missing from the syllabus or, if mentioned, are only in conjunction with lectures on aspects of kidney disease, yet 10 per cent of a doctor's time in general practice is taken up with women's urinary infections. The medical schools are out of touch with the common, simple medical complaints of life and, I believe, often fail their young trainee doctors. High-tech medicine is all the rage, so are more 'unique' illnesses that do not affect so many thousands of patients. Most of us want the illnesses that affect the majority of people to be cured in simple, effective ways. Instead millions of pounds are poured into new engineering that may help only a handful of people.

When I lecture to a medical audience, I do like to quote the following figures from a 1972 survey in which the then members of the U & I (Urinary Infection/You and I) Club participated; 750 answers were received.

Q. How many cystoscopies have you had?

A. 774 (between the 750 women)
Q. Have you needed further major renal surgery?
A. 50 out of the 750 women needed operations or treatment

So time and money had in effect been wasted on the remaining 724 women. That time and money could have been used for all manner of other medical help.

Why did the doctors do this?

Answer:

They had not been taught effective alternatives.

Medical interference is costly and, in the case of urinary infection, unnecessary and ineffective. The quality of your life in this regard is entirely within your own hands. It is so for millions of women around the world like you.

Personal Hygiene

In many countries, women practise differing methods of hygiene, and many as a result suffer fewer urinary problems than we in Britain do. Female hygiene and bladder care is in the hands of the bladder's owner – you!

Over the years of preaching this gospel I have used two methods of washing away the bacteria that cause urinary infections.

The earlier one worked for some extra-careful women. It was not at all foolproof. The latest, called *bottle washing*, is 100 per cent foolproof for all women, no matter what their social or financial circumstances, if they do it correctly.

Having said that, it can instantly be qualified! There are many countries where clean water is absent. Clean water is central to hygiene and good health. We may not like the taste of big city tap water, but compared with the water of, say, Calcutta or Lagos it is superb and, what's more:

- there's enough of it
- it is piped into our own homes
- we can make it hot or cold
- it is largely uncontaminated

We do not value it as we should. When you have to wash your whole body in one basin of water, twice a week, you quickly learn to value it, I can tell you!

As many of my readers will know, I learned this fact in Lagos, Nigeria. It was at this time I also stopped washing my perineum with a flannel. From my first week in Lagos I adopted the brilliant method of bottle washing.

The tap water in our home, like everywhere else in Lagos, was brown and gritty. Within three days I had my first urinary infection in four years despite maintaining my normal rigorous hygiene procedures.

The only thing different was the quality of the tap water. So, watching my stewards each day filtering and boiling this brown liquid and then storing it in old orange drink bottles in the fridge to use for cleaning vegetables, making ice, etc., I found another use for it. Two more bottles were prepared and put beside the lavatory in my bathroom.

From that day, in September 1976, I have had only one brief urinary infection (in June 1987).

Bottle Washing

Faecal material – that is, what your stools are composed of – is greasy. Even when you use masses of lavatory paper you can never remove the microscopic bacterial faecal residue.

Think of a frying pan. You can wipe it dry with a whole roll of kitchen paper but it will still smell and be covered with a thin, invisible film of grease.

The invisible residue of your faecal bacteria left on your perineum after a bowel movement is the direct bacterial source which gives rise to your urinary infections. As you walk around, the backwards and forwards movements of your legs spread the bacterial residue along the length of the perineum to the vulval area.

Certain extra circumstances help a continued journey of the germs into the urethral opening and up into the bladder.

Those circumstances are:

- poor perineal hygiene
- sexual intercourse
- catheters
- old and thin vulval skin
- physical disabilities or injury
- haemorrhoids
- episiotomy scars
- diarrhoea
- stiff or arthritic limbs

There are lots of other individual extras which vary from woman to woman. Nevertheless, their damage can be avoided by bottle washing.

First let's take a look at a couple of the circumstances listed above to see exactly how they contribute to urinary infection.

Sexual Intercourse
This is the commonest way for coliform and other faecal bacteria to be helped into the bladder. As intercourse takes place the urethra and bladder, which lie alongside the vagina, are virtually pummelled by the friction. Faecal residue thus gets massaged into the urethral tube and into the vaginal entrance. Once coliforms are introduced into the mildly acidic, moist urethra they continue to breed at a tremendous rate. Coliforms divide every 20 minutes! Just imagine then, if you passed a

stool at 10 a.m. and had intercourse at 10 p.m., what a colony you would have on your perineum! And that colony would be more than ready to overspill into urethral territory with the help of sexual activity.

Oral intercourse of any kind transmits bacteria to and from each partner. Urinary symptoms in such circumstances are different from an attack of cystitis. They may be general malaise, kidney pain, bladder disturbance, occasional bladder twingeing or bladder soreness. Often the bacteria responsible are not sought out in ordinary labs and suffering continues apace with any old antibiotic or none being prescribed because samples are repeatedly negative. Bacteria in smegma under the foreskin can be: urea plasma, Haemophilus Influenzae, mixed anaerobes and aerobes from dental diseases, Tuberculosis, Streptococcus Pneumoniae, Moraxella Catarrhalis, Streptococcus Group F from sinus, throat and mouth infections as well as the usual Staphs and Streps. More unusual anal bacteria coming from the gut and anal sexual transfer may include Tuberculosis, Citrobacter, Staphs and Streps, any of the coliforms and more. Oral sexual contact inevitably means that much bacteria is swallowed, digested and colonises in the kidneys. Bacterial drip into the bloodstream influences the whole system causing pain and frequency. Do not have any oral sex unless both partners have washed carefully beforehand.

Old and Thin Vulval Skin

All skin ages. From 45 years old it ages faster because the female hormone levels decrease. Skin, internally as well as externally, becomes wrinkly and crinkly. The cells that make up a balanced, healthy padding start to break down, as does their efficiency at throwing off bacterial attacks.

Stiff or Arthritic Limbs

In older age, women get stiffer. They cannot bend so easily and some quite old women cannot bathe or wash as well as they used to. They may not even be quite able to use loo paper properly. Older women need their urine tested reasonably often to spot higher sugar levels, which could denote early signs of diabetes. Coliforms and other faecal bacteria love a diet of sugar, and diabetes provides exactly that. So, in the mildly acidic urine, sugar is an added growth factor. Hormone Replacement Therapy (HRT) can go some way to reverse this process.

How to Wash Effectively

A bath a day for sufferers from urinary infections is no good, for two reasons:

1. You may not be bathing immediately after passing a stool – thereby leaving the perineum contaminated indefinitely.
2. If you do bath afterwards you will be sitting in a solution of bacteria.

Showering is a little better than bathing, but again is useless unless done straight away, which can be inconvenient.

The timing of when you wash cannot be stressed too firmly. If you bath or shower at 7.45 a.m. and pass a stool *afterwards*, that bacterial residue remains until 7.45 the next morning.

It is far better if you pass a stool at 7.44 a.m. and bath or shower at 7.45; the bacterial residue will now be washed off.

However, even showering at the right time is not foolproof, because of the way the water drips off the gravity point on the perineum. Standing straight allows shower water to drip off *all along* the perineum, which means that bacterial residue can run forwards to the vagina. Buttocks are generally tense in a slippery shower, which means that water may or may not run backwards cleanly over the back passage opening. I don't advise it as a foolproof perineal cleaning process.

Bottle Washing

Done precisely, bottle washing is 100 per cent effective, quick, costs nothing and can be done anywhere at all, at virtually any time, unless you are in the bushes somewhere! Remember these 'three Bs' in precise order: *1. Bowels, 2. Bottle, 3. Bath*

I am going to explain the bottle washing method point by point, for use when your are at home, at work, or out. Then I will describe the method point by point for bottle washing the vagina after sex, to reduce bruising or infection, and for cleaning out annoying discharges while you are waiting for swab results.

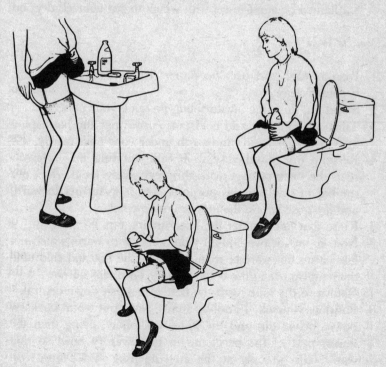

Figure 11: Bottle washing

Procedure I

Bottle Washing After Passing a Stool at Home
For those with an 'all-in' bathroom i.e. lavatory and hand-basin in one room.
You require:

- a basin
- a lavatory, well cleaned
- one or two 500-ml (1-pint/20 fl. oz) tonic/soda bottles
  – not larger or smaller
- a bar of non-perfumed, non-medicated, non-deodorized soap
- a flannel or guest towel with which to pat yourself dry

Now, to Work!

1. Pass a stool and use loo paper (from behind) until this becomes clean.
2. Stand up, flush the lavatory but *don't* pull your pants up.
3. Turn on both hot and cold taps – *don't* put the basin plug in. Wash your hands and scrub under your nails briefly.
4. Re-soap one hand very well. Still standing up, *thoroughly* soap the back passage with this very soapy hand. *Don't* use the bar of soap for this purpose, *don't* soap further forward, and *don't* use wipes, flannels or cotton wool.
5. Rinse that hand under the hot, running tap. No plug!
6. Now fill one or two 500-ml soda bottles with warm water, not lukewarm, but warmer than that. Mix the hot and cold until the temperature in the bottle is right. Turn taps off now.
7. Return to the toilet with the bottle(s) and sit down centrally.
8. Position yourself, buttocks apart. Now put your back*bone* down (pelvic tilt) and the anus will follow, being then the lowest part of the perineum in the lavatory bowl so that water falls off only at the anal opening and cannot run uphill to the vaginal opening.

9. *From the front*, pour the warm bottle of water between your legs. You must use your other hand to clean the labia and then reach downwards to help clear away completely *all* traces of the soap which now contains all the bacteria. Use the second bottle if all the soap hasn't gone. When the soap is off, so are the bacteria.

10. Stand up and pat the perineum dry with the flannel or small guest towel. Keep this apart on its own hook, even though there aren't any germs on it. They are down the loo.

Remember, faecal material is greasy. It will only come off with warm water *and* soap!

Common Mistakes in Bottle Washing

- Not enough soap
- Using bottles that are too big or too small, or milk bottles that should have been sterilized, or jugs that pour badly. *Only* use 500 ml soda bottles; they have been carefully chosen and researched.
- Not sitting on the loo with anus as the lowest point.
- Leaning back against the lavatory cistern. You just can't reach the back passage from this position and the seat clenches the buttocks, preventing water from a clear backward flow.
- Using cotton wool or a flannel to put the soap on with. Don't! You contaminate yourself, block up the loo, and will miss the skin folds and any haemorrhoids. Only apply soap with your hand so that all nooks and crannies get soapy.
- Using a bidet. A bidet is dangerous, it spreads bacteria around.
- Putting the basin plug in and rinsing your hands in a solution of faecal bacteria.
- Not doing it every time you open your bowels and think-

ing that missing it once will be all right! Just you dare!

- Standing in the bath with one leg on the edge and trying to shower the perineum.
- Squatting in the bath – just plain difficult, dangerous and unnecessary.
- Sitting on the edge of the bath instead of the lavatory.
- Pouring the bottle from behind so that faecal germs run forward.

Procedure II

Bottle Washing for Those with a Separate Loo and Bathroom
You will need the same 'equipment' as for Procedure I.

1. Pass a stool and use loo paper until it comes clean. Flush the pan.
2. Go into the bathroom and wash your hands well.
3. Leaving the hot tap running, re-soap one hand and soap the back passage very well with it.
4. Rinse that hand under the running hot tap.
5. Now fill *both* 500-ml bottles with warm/hot water.
6. Walk from your bathroom into your lavatory.
7. Proceed as from Procedure I, point 7 until point 10.
11. Return the two bottles to the bathroom ready for next time.

Procedure III

Bottle Washing at Work
This is designed for those of you who pass a stool regularly at work, and who have a desk or a locker for personal possessions.

When you buy the 500-ml bottles for use at home, buy two more for work. Also buy a toilet bag that will hold the two bottles, a kitchen paper roll and soap, to leave at your work-place.

1. Take the equipped toilet bag with you to the rest room.
2. First wash your hands *very* well and then fill the two 500-ml bottles with very warm water.
3. Break off a couple of pieces of kitchen roll, fold in half, pass them once through the hot water tap and soap both of them. Do not use toilet paper; it disintegrates.
4. Go into the lavatory cubicle. Put both bottles down some-where – perhaps on the floor or a ledge on another piece of kitchen roll. Lodge the two soaped pieces of kitchen roll somewhere clean, e.g. next to the bottles on a piece of kitchen roll.
5. Line the loo seat with loo paper, sit down and pass a stool. Use loo paper as usual.
6. Pick up the soaped kitchen roll pieces and, still sitting, though leaning forward a bit more, soap the back passage well with each piece. Drop them down the loo behind you.
7. Now re-position yourself so that the back passage is lowest in the pan as per Procedure I, point 8.
8. Pour the bottled warm water down the perineum from the front, using your spare hand to clean away all traces of soap. Use the second bottle if necessary.
9. Break off two more pieces of kitchen roll and *dab* the peri-neum dry. If you don't dab you may get minute particles of paper left on the perineum. Kitchen roll is less likely to leave particles than toilet paper.
10. Wash hands at the basin and take the toilet bag back to your desk or locker.
11. Remember to remove the loo paper lining the lavatory seat and to leave the loo in a respectable state.

Always refer back to Procedure I if you are in any doubt about the steps involved.

Should you run out of kitchen roll and forget to bring in more, you can use those green paper towels that are sometimes provided by a wall dispenser – but *don't block the loo*. If your cleaning procedure has been less than adequately done, repeat as soon as you are home.

Procedure IV

Bottle Washing for Those 'Caught Short'
This is also the method to use if your place of work does not accommodate Procedure III.

The rules bend a great deal here. The one aim is only to do your best. Those green towels may have to do for both the soaping and the rinsing, but such attempts are purely temporary. Full bottle washing must be done when you arrive home. *Never* have sexual intercourse if you have had a bowel movement that day and have not washed afterwards. If you are sexually active it is vital to bottle wash fully in advance of intercourse. If you have passed wind which contains faecal bacteria, as we all do, this must be washed off *before* sex

You see, it is the downward, backward flow of water which successfully removes the soap and deposits the bacteria in the lavatory pan water. Everything else is less effective, probably even wrong.

So, recognizing that fact, I will still run through this procedure point by point for those of you needing emergency washing.

1. Go to the basins first if you are in a strange rest room.
2. Check the green towel situation. If there are none, abandon the idea of washing until you get home.
or
3. Check your handbag for paper hankies: got some? Four will do.
4. Wash your hands very well.

5. So, with either green towels or four paper hankies, pass one green towel (they are quite thick) under the hot tap and then soap it a little. fold it up again. Alternatively, soap each of two paper hankies, which are less strong.
6. Now wet the remainder, to be used for rinsing.
7. Go to the lavatory, then proceed as for Procedure III, point 5 until you get to point 8; *then,*
8. Still leaning forward, wipe the back passage from behind, pulling the green towel or paper hankies away and backwards. Fold over and wipe again until all traces of soap have gone.

I personally am quite good at this when I have to be. Just follow logic, get the soap off and remember, you can (and should) fully bottle wash back home in an hour or so's time.

Men who fail to use sufficient toilet paper effectively wipe their faecal residue all over their underwear. Depending on whether they position genitalia within underwear, also whether tight jeans or trousers cause sweating, so this faecal residue can be transferred in intercourse.

Check out their underwear and towels (your own also) for faecal staining. Men never use enough toilet paper and often do not soap or clean the anal opening in the shower or bath.

Men and women should use lots of soap on the anal opening. *In the shower*, water will follow gravity and can run forwards into the urethral and vaginal openings. Last thing, face the shower and clean off all soapy residue from either vulva (in women) or penis. *In the bath*, clean and rinse the anus last thing. Stand up to soap it then sit for a moment. Finally, stand again and shower off the whole perineum from front to back.

Other Risky Factors

So you are an ordinary woman with an ordinary bowel movement. I was, once! Now I am older and the mother of two children, with the results of my labours showing clearly upon my perineum! To wit, one episiotomy scar and one smallish group of external skin tabs. They are not proper haemorrhoids but the skin no longer sits on the anal orifice as it did in my youthful pre-pregnancy years.

I don't get diarrhoea or loose bowels except if I have a tummy bug, but for many women diarrhoea and irritable bowels can be daily scourges.

Episiotomy Scars

These are miserable. I don't honestly know what's worse: a cut from anus to vagina to shorten a long, strained labour, or a long, strained labour in which pelvic floor muscles lose elasticity and give rise in later years to a prolapsed uterus or a prolapsed bladder.

This episiotomy scar never goes. Every act of intercourse, every bowel strain adds up to further stress and ageing upon it. The long line of the scar tissue has less resistance to the movement of bacteria upon it and, as I have said before, it becomes a railway for fast bacterial travel.

It is another aid to a dose of urinary infection.

Haemorrhoids or Skin Tabs

These are common upon the female anal orifice. Young girls can get them if the consistency of stools is very hard; women in pregnancy suffer from them; older women get them from years spent standing up for long periods of time; and really old women get them from sitting down all day.

Depending upon your circumstances, it will pay to have your doctor inject the haemorrhoids with anti-inflammatory liquid to shrink the swellings and to prevent a worsening of the situation. The procedure is uncomfortable but not really painful. You may need some rest and painkillers afterwards, but you will feel better next day. The results are usually very good and lasting.

Maybe the haemorrhoids are bad enough to consider operating and removing, or maybe you only need to change your breakfast cereal and stop sugar to encourage looser stools. Suppositories and creams may help temporarily, but if you get to the point of needing these every day, forever, then it might be time to have the haemorrhoids injected.

Irregular and disturbed levels of anal skin provides nooks and crannies in which residual faecal bacteria multiply. Haemorrhoids are a common factor in repeated urinary infections.

Diarrhoea and Irritable Bowels

Well, these things happen in all age groups and for a million reasons. What counts, yet again, in preventing cystitis is whether you wash off that residual faecal bacteria after a bowel movement.

Obviously, if you can sort out the reasons for the upset bowel, you should, but you'll be passing a stool every day even if you *do* improve the bowel's activity. You must wash after *every* bowel motion all your life. The undertakers are going to do me!

Having impressed all these points clearly upon you, what follows are the procedures for bottle washing after sex or for washing out discharge from the vagina.

Procedure V

Bottle Washing After Sex

This simple washing must *only* be done *after* a full bottle washing as per Procedure I. If you attempt to do it on an unclean perineum you could introduce faecal bacteria to the vagina and cervix.

So – after sex, to clean out sexual liquids that could irritate the vagina and perineum next day, get up and go into the bathroom and:

1. First, wash your hands.
2. Fill up the one or two 500-ml soda bottles with *cool* water this time, which will help to reduce swelling and soreness.
3. Sit on the lavatory and pass urine.
4. Re-position yourself until the anus is the lowest part of you in the lavatory bowl (pelvic tilt).
5. Pour the *cool* bottled water slowly down the labia and put the longest finger of your spare hand into the vagina. Water will enter with it.
6. When the finger comes out, sexual liquid will, too, in the water.
7. Keep repeating this action until the vagina feels nice and clean again. Five or six times should do the job.
8. Pour a last swill of cool water down the entire perineum and then pat quite dry with your flannel or guest towel.

The flannel is much the best and, because it is only for drying (there are no germs on it), I put it in with the other laundry every five days. If you know that your skin is sensitive to washing powders then don't do this. Boil it up in an old saucepan instead.

Cool water reduces sexual bruising and is a wonderful healer of inflamed skin. You will also have noticed that no soap is used in this procedure. Never use soap frontally; the liquids and moisture of the vagina, vulva and urethra are non-greasy. Only fae-cal bacteria is greasy enough to *need* the soap routine of Procedure I. In fact, soap used at the front usually causes many a dose of cystitis from sensitive skin reactions, no matter what soap you use. I must again stress that perineal preparation *before* intercourse is the only way to stop bacterial sexual cystitis. Sex occurs and cystitis starts from the perineal con-ditions *during* sex, not when it is all over. Remember; *Perineum Preparatum!*

One more general tip: On no account be tempted to use per-fumed, deodorized, coloured or antiseptic soaps on the perineum – elsewhere OK, but not on the perineum.

You might want to make a copy of the Procedure instruc-tions and pin it up in the bathroom or lavatory for a few days until you get it precisely right.

Bottle washing takes only 20 to 30 seconds to do after you have passed a stool, that's all. It is designed not only to be 100 per cent effective in preventing infections but also to be quick. It is quicker than doing your teeth once you do it as I instruct. Don't think that you know better than me, just accept that after years of research and success, I know better than you! I have also been free of trouble for nearly 20 years, by following my own instructions.

Lingering Bacteria

If recurrent attacks seem now to have rolled into one continu-ous twinge every day of every week, the bottle washing will stop all new incoming faecal bacteria. However, old pockets of inflammation or even bacteria can linger. We must look after the internal side of this as well, so:

1. Drink a glass of water every two hours and also pass urine then. Drink and void.

2. Take painkillers to calm the upset bladder nerve impulses – say first thing in the morning and last thing at night.

3. Take Cymalon, Cystopurin or potassium citrate (as instructed on the packet directions or by your pharmacist) to decrease any acidity. Potter's 'Antitis' (UK brand name) is also helpful.

4. A course of multi-minerals will help the immune system responses.

5. If all is no better after two months, have a three-day course of antibiotics. Keep the self-help going and take further sporadic courses of antibiotics if necessary.

6. I have known severe inflammation to take six months to decrease in some women. Any increase in comfort levels should be seen as a good sign.

7. Check out the vagina for any trouble there causing secondary urethral symptoms.

Finally

Everyone leads a different life, has different standards of medical care, differing symptoms and differing resources with which to combat problems. I am always willing to counsel anyone still in difficulties, so don't keep suffering. You might find my video, for example, very helpful. If you want to contact me for any reason, write to the address given at the back of this book.

Part 2

NON-BACTERIAL CYSTITIS

Chapter 6

JUST CHATTING

Medical Obstacles

If roughly 60 per cent of all cases of cystitis are caused by
bowel germs travelling to and setting up an attack in the bladder, then roughly 40 per cent are caused by something else.
This 'something else' can be very simple or it can be a whole
parcel of problems that needs unravelling in stages, patiently. It
is at this point that the medical profession flaps its hands and
finds fashionable phrases such as 'Urethral Syndrome' or
'Interstitial Cystitis'.

To unravel patiently is seldom entirely the task set for the
sufferer alone. Often, medical investigations and complicity are
very important; often the parcel has been constructed in the
first place by medical mishap or ignorance, with the patient
bowing to 'the powers that be' in the doctor's surgery or hospital. There are two rules to remember when dealing with
medical bureaucracy: first, never agree to surgical intervention
unless you have had a second opinion or been for knowledgeable counselling and lengthy discussion, and secondly, keep
searching for the causes of your cystitis.

There are many other areas of medicine upon which bladder

and urinary problems impinge but practitioners nevertheless tend to stick rigidly to the boundaries of their particular speciality. Most obviously and still commonly, for example, a gynaecologist will seldom discuss or investigate urinary problems and a urologist will be reluctant to examine the vagina or bowels. Yet it is only too clear that different conditions constantly intermingle within a woman's body.

Those patients coming to me for counselling with this 'parcel' usually have a couple of extra problems which may prevent a happy outcome, even when they follow my suggestions:

1. The quality of care where they live may already be a difficulty. In addition, their doctor's or hospital's knowledge and support may be lacking, leaving these women with no remaining options.
2. They may lack the funds necessary to pursue other options outside the NHS. I recommend that all women should have private health insurance or should talk to their bank manager about a loan to cover such expenses.

I quite agree that the NHS should be perfectly able to help – after all, millions are spent on high-tech operations in terms of both time and resources in order to help a handful of people, so why can't urology and gynaecology take time to pursue treatment of the greater number of sufferers whose problems, over time, eat away at precious funding?

Just 'going private' is not an infallible key to success. It all still depends upon a particular doctor's knowledge and training. His or her experience with cystitis victims counts a great deal; a 'feel' for the difficulties, a 'hunch' played out and a real understanding of all the interlinking conditions. Everyone involved must be sure of the cause, or causes, and suggestions or treatments only then should be advised.

Taking A Case History

The medical idea of how to take case history is not the same as my idea of taking one. Mine, of course, also starts with name and address, etc., but then, before any symptoms are taken down, I want to know a lot about a woman's social and work background. Has she a husband/partner? What is his job/hobbies? What does the sufferer do for a living/hobby? I also like to find out about a woman's hours of work, her age, children, details of her home and much more, depending upon her answers as we go along. This question/answer probing provides important diagnostic details.

Then I'll ask about her symptoms, when they started, when they come, the day, week or month, any patterns she has noticed, tests she has had done so far, MSU results, operations, and on it goes. Some women can be with me for two and a half hours, some for one if it is a follow-up. Women come from all over Britain, and beyond. Most are desperate, of course, and all go away with a list of ideas and suggestions. It can be a short list or it can run to many points. I don't examine or prescribe, but the difference made when my ideas and suggestions have been put into practice can be quite dramatic. No doctor anywhere has the time or instincts for this approach. It isn't alternative medicine – it is logic and common sense most of the time, and a bit of detective work.

Pioneering

Two historical figures in particular have had similar approaches. The first was Ignaz Philip Semmelweiss, a Hungarian Jewish obstetrician practising in Budapest. He began to wonder why, of the two delivery wards in his hospital, his ward had the higher of the heavy maternity death rates. The midwives on the other ward did better. Why? After much research and heartbreak, he came to the idea that it might have something to do with his medical students, who rather than trained midwives did the deliveries on his ward. He knew that these students would always proceed directly to the delivery ward after carving up dead, putrid bodies in the dissecting room. The midwives weren't allowed in the dissecting room!

Remember, bacteria were unknown in the mid-18th century. By accident he discovered that when he washed his own hands before assisting at a birth, the mother tended not to die! He introduced a bowl of water and soap at the door of the ward and placed a guard on hand to insist that everyone washed before entering. The death rate began to fall and puerperal fever began to decline over the next century.

Florence Nightingale wasn't so much a pioneer in fighting one specific illness as in the fight against the many conditions surrounding illness which tended to exacerbate it and/or its victim's suffering. She was a great believer in hope, reassurance, cleanliness and a preventative approach to illnesses. Environment, both in hospitals and at home, was to her mind very important. She well knew the value of effective sewerage and clean available water. Knowledgeable, kindly nursing was all a part of her ethos.

Both these excellent people had to take a softly, softly approach with their contemporaries. Both had setbacks and scepticism to deal with, yet they were so right and now their work is an integral part of all modern medicine. My own work tries to follow their example. Correct hygiene and common sense are my cornerstones, too. This must be kept up. When you get well, you must tell your doctors and put this book in front of them.

No More Desperation

Only since 1942 have sufferers from cystitis avoided dying. Women everywhere, until the last 50 years or so, became extremely ill and frequently died from urinary problems. Usually it was the rising *E. coli* infections lodging for months at a time in the kidneys, whose working efficiency was impaired as a result. The two World Wars, especially the Second, saw wounds and venereal diseases killing as many off the battle-ground as on it. Luckily, Alexander Fleming discovered peni-cillin and so, with the birth of antibiotics, a revolution was brought about in the treatment of infection anywhere in the human body. Kidney disease caused by the rising coliforms was hugely decreased and antibiotic therapy remains the com-monest medical response to cystitis.

Antibiotics, as useful as they are, should only be prescribed if infection is proven – but sympathy for the patient, together with her acceptance of 'anything' that will help, usually leads to a course of antibiotics being prescribed anyway. First-aid management of attacks and the many non-bacterial causes of attacks, however, render them (as a sole method of treatment) unacceptable.

Non-Bacterial Cystitis: A Case History

Jane had twingeing by the end of each working day, leading sometimes to attacks of full-blown frequency pain and bleeding when she passed urine. She was a hard pressed personal assis-tant to a frenetic company chairman. No bacteria was ever found in samples. The trouble began when she started in this job and she was more comfortable at weekends – vital diag-nostic clues. Her drinking habits ceased to exist after breakfast except for a cold coffee when she could remember and a glass of wine at lunch if she managed a break. Around 3.00 p.m., time permitting, she had a cup of tea.

No bladder could function with this routine; water is required to dilute the acids and to stop crystals gathering in the urethral tube. Increasing her water intake stopped all her symptoms; antibiotics that had never helped had been proven not necessary and now didn't need to be taken even out of desperation.

This is one of thousands of individual reasons for non-bacterial cystitis. Yet every one of the individual reasons ever found can fall into one of the following categories:

- dehydration
- irritation
- chemical contamination
- clothing
- lifestyle in general

Over the next five chapters each of these reasons will be examined, and you will learn how to prevent them from leading to cystitis. Remember: women cause their own cystitis unwittingly. What follows will give you the wits to stop it.

Chapter 7

DEHYDRATION

Exploitation of Water

The most precious life-sustaining substance on the planet is water. Wars are fought over it and territory mapped out to include access to rivers and seas. It represented the earliest means of long-distance travel, and irrigation canals have been cut into great dry areas allowing more food to be locally grown.

All living plants and creatures need water for cell preservation and blood bulk. As humans we have many pints of it in our bodies at any one time – as 'capital', if you like; we also require a 'cash flow' of it. It is the cash flow on a daily level that dictates the health of our kidneys, bladder and urethra. We cannot clean *them* as we can the perineum with physical contact; we can only do so by eating and drinking sensibly: caring for them as they require.

Our diet and liquid intake have evolved from the simplest food and drink sources. Cave people ate berries, greenery, fish and red meats and drank only water and milk until the process of mixing fermented fruits led to the discovery of alcohol. We progressed, learning to work with all sorts of climates and locations to yield popular, staple foods. Life remained fairly simple. Of course, people were often ill from lack of hygiene and gut parasites from eating infected animals, but this became more controllable in the 19th and 20th centuries. Mass food production for town dwellers meant developing ways of preserving food all the way from the farm to the shop shelf and larder.

These days we are becoming concerned about the methods employed to harvest and prepare our food and drink – about insecticides and additives. We have to face a bewildering array of choice, all the while trying to read every label to find out exactly what is in the food we are buying. Even if we could understand the list of contents on food packaging, reading them all is a ridiculously time-consuming effort. So we don't always bother.

Our understanding of liquid intake is very blurred nowadays as well. We need water to top up our cash flow, but on offer are tea, coffee, fruit juices, canned drinks, alcoholic beverages, milk and many others. Liquid can also be taken up in meals, stews, roasts, salads, vegetables, fruits; in tinned foods, frozen or fresh. But the actual glass of water is the caring, kind and best way to keep kidneys, bladder and urethra at their happiest and healthiest.

- The caffeine in tea, coffee, sweet drinks, etc. is a kidney stimulant.
- Diuretics, which can be found in many foods and drinks, especially alcohol, again encourage a fast output from the kidneys.
- Stress or fear can make adrenaline surge, again stimulating the kidneys.
- Drinking excessively will make the kidneys and bladder speed up and excrete the excess that cannot be used by cells and organs.

Gullibility

All drinks are made attractive to the shopper. The packaging is a researched, state of the art exercise inviting the shopper to reach out and take it off the shelf. It is not just one item either, because the more you buy, the better a deal you'll be offered:

'Buy 10, get the 11th free!'

'Buy 2 packs and the 3rd is free!'

Buying in bulk can make sense for some products, if you have the storage space, but this hype is all just a sales gimmick. The company needs to make money. Nothing wrong in that, but it should depend on the honesty and validity of the product. Children in particular are heavily targeted by the marketing departments of, for example, the major fizzy drinks companies. Fizzy pops are often all that many of these gullible children drink, and so parental or school control is left to fight the results: energized, addictive, hyperactive children.

Colas, fruit juices, coffee and alcohol are all loaded with sugars, additives and diuretics. They can cause heavy urinary output, making the kidneys process the volumes involved at high speed. For young kidneys, this extra work on a daily basis is detrimental to their health, and continues to be so for the rest of their lives.

Is Drinking Water Safe?

Some time ago, I went down with *Giardia*, a water-borne parasite that exists normally in most countries' water supplies, including those of Russia, Eastern Europe and parts of Western Europe. The UK has seen several outbreaks of the condition caused by this parasite. It is hard to diagnose, but makes you very unwell, with explosive wind and diarrhoea several times a day. I drank it unknowingly in Germany, scoffing at the offered bottled waters. It took three months to diagnose and nine months to treat, since the antibiotics most usually prescribed simply failed to effect lasting relief. Treatment with a homoeopathic drug called Paramesis stopped my symptoms 24 hours later, but eradicating the complete infestation took many weeks, and had to be accompanied by close attention to my diet – no red meat and not a drop of coffee or alcohol.

The episode shook me up considerably. My feelings of high regard for German standards changed to utter dismay when I learned that drinking water there is, by and large, infested with parasites of all kinds. What's more, isolated parasite infestations of UK water supplies are now occurring, with more expected as travel between countries increases. I feel very saddened and worried about the prospect of unusable tap water in the UK. It is already filled with cleansing chemicals and even so is often barely above recommended safety levels. A strong resilient gut is needed to overcome possible reactions to these cleansers, yet at the same time no one wants a return to the days of yore when the water was so infested everyone had worms and parasites.

I have given in and now only drink bottled waters, though I will still use tap water boiled for hot drinks. One Christmas my son gave me a simple tap water filter jug with a replaceable filter cartridge. Twelve days later my sensitive system went under to the chemicals and silver used to cleanse and filter the water. I became weak, dizzy and had strong stomach pains even after only one mouthful. My tap water is in any case usable, so it was back to that and bottled mineral water. Water, clean water, is simply the most vital element necessary for staying alive and healthy.

Capital Savings and Cash Flow

The point at which our bodies reach dehydration can vary. Account must be taken of weather conditions (hot or cold), sweating, fevers, exercise, certain illnesses, alcohol intake, whether we even want to drink. I know women who aren't in the habit of drinking. They just can't be bothered. They are too busy or they forget. Full dehydration, a level rarely reached except in cases drought or in those with chronic diarrhoea, can lead to death. The kidneys draw upon the contents of other cells and organs to help them continue filtering impurities out of the blood. Finally, when such capital supplies are exhausted, kidney function ceases. The end result of continuous diuretic activity is lowered body liquid levels. The natural inclination then to feel thirsty is the body's effort to balance and replace these lost liquids for its own good.

Failure to drink sufficient amounts of water creates a continuously lower level at which the kidneys cannot work. Without enough, they cannot dilute the urine which carries impurities, such as acids and enzymes which have completed their tasks in the kidneys. These can be very strong if undiluted.

Bladder Function and Reaction

Rejected substances all flow in urine down a tube from each kidney called a ureter. Gravity propels droplets every few seconds towards a valve which will only open when a certain amount of urine has gathered behind it. This liquid weight then makes the valve open to allow it through, directly into the bladder. The bladder is a receptacle for storing urine. It has no other function. Why then can it be such a painful and problem-prone organ?

It is painful because without exceptional sensitivity it wouldn't know when it was full. Exploding isn't one of nature's aims, so fail-safe methods of preventing explosion are essential! Nerve endings in the bladder are virtually surface-based and super-responsive. What we put into our digestive system and what we allow up into the bladder via the urethra from outside are major influences governing many bladder problems.

If the bladder receives the results of a night's bar drinking, it must open and expel as often as it fills up. This can mean many trips to the bathroom. If it receives an invasion of bacteria from the urethral opening, its natural response is to try and eject the problem. If you get a fever from a virus or infection, the bladder's reaction (to excrete and expel the toxins) are part of the body's defence mechanism. In addition to these come all manner of situations that set up reactions.

Not drinking enough may well stop the bladder's regular activity of five or six openings a day, but the crystallization of the bladder lining and urethral lining, brought on by insufficient fluids, can lead to trouble. Without a regular flow over these areas to keep them moist and prevent crystal deposits, crystal formation (which isn't just the uric acid, but also the many filtered toxins and waste products that pass through the bladder and urethral tubes) can settle and adhere to these sensitive surfaces. Inflammation begins.

Once begun, the contents of the crystals, now in contact with super-sensitive nerve endings, will activate defence mechanisms. Mild twingeing, spasms and shudders will become apparent and the bathroom beckons. So then you pass a small, dark quantity, which may or may not hurt, like a cystitis attack, and could leave you feeling as though you need to go again soon after. Much of this and inflammation proper can lead to an increase in the twingeing, sufficient to make you think you have proper cystitis.

Sensible Drinking

Think back over the past few days. Have you drunk the suggested 3–4 pints (60–80 fl. oz/1.5–2 litres) of the day's kidney liquid cash flow? Perhaps you have, but perhaps your body has required even more liquid than normal of late. Have you been working out, have you gone dancing, do you have a cold, have you been rushing around at work, have you had lengthy sex, eaten a Chinese meal with lots of monosodium glutamate (or MSG, a salty additive used in many Chinese dishes), taken a plane trip, got cold at the bus stop, drunk too much coffee? The list is endless because all of us lead different lives, but such factors can, for many women, make the difference between twingeing and comfort.

Listen to what your body dictates. Drink if you feel thirsty. Drink regularly anyway. Don't let crystals and acidity compromise your urinary system. Dehydration in all its forms is hazardous, and failure to empty the bladder at reasonable intervals is careless.

Drink and void (empty) are essential rules for cystitis-prone people.

'Not Quite Right'

If you have found the basic reason/s for your attacks of cystitis but you can still tell that things are 'not quite right', the chances are that remaining patches of inflamed skin, either in the bladder or urethra, are still sore. Internal healing can take a while. Some women recover quickly, others slowly; some so slowly that recovery is unnoticeable for the first weeks. Sometimes it can be helpful to have kept a 'journal' of symptoms, etc. I use one with the women I counsel; in a return visit with a woman's previous notes in front of me I can point to differences between her current state and what it was like before. Listing off the changes can be uplifting and morale-boosting. Patience can be renewed and hope once again encouraged.

Sometimes adjustments, fine tuning, in the already improving circumstances can make quite a leap in further symptom reduction.

Joanna had come for counselling on her attacks of cystitis, which had regularly ruined her new sexual relationship. We had sorted it all out and she'd had her first sexual holiday in three years. Her slight remaining problem was that passing urine afterwards often didn't 'produce' urine. In order to reduce sexual bruising, I always recommend that the bowels be opened daily and that a full bladder be emptied before sex. This she was happy to comply with, but often sex was short – about half-an-hour, and afterwards, when she went to the loo, there wasn't enough urine ready to be voided. Since most of the sex was occurring at night, the 8 to 10 hours or so of sleep that followed until 7.30 or 8.00 next morning made that next, early morning excretion a bit sorer than she was happy with.

I helped her to 'fine-tune' it. I advised her that, when she passed urine before sex, either to leave some behind or have a drink beforehand. This would enable more after-sex excretion, as indeed it did. No matter how little is passed, it must be passed to de-traumatize the 'shocked' bladder and get it settled. A small glass of water after sex does help the early morning urine excretion to be paler or more comfortable. Sex uses up a lot of energy. Sweating, orgasms and natural vaginal lubrication all help remove cell liquid and excite the kidneys. Replace the lost liquids and restore urinary balance, or cystitis, effectively from dehydration, may start.

Check List for Dehydration

If you think that the cause of your sort of cystitis could be due to poor liquid intake, check it out with as much proof as you can find.

1. Have you drunk three pints today, at reasonably regular intervals? One or two heavy liquid sessions is not a regular,

gentle input. Such sessions in themselves overwork the kidneys and excess is simply sent straight to the bladder. Some liquid needs to be allocated for cell and organ storage, as well as for urine bulk. Downing liquid in a heavy 'cash flow' session won't allow for this as efficiently as regular small amounts.

2. Are your urine samples always negative? Of course, there are mountainous reasons for negative results as well as dehydration, but you still need to know that the cystitis is definitely non-bacterial.

3. Do twinges seem to start towards midday or late afternoon? Maybe they are constant? This can mean intake is too low during the morning or afternoon. Often sensations decrease once a woman is at home and drinking sensibly. Teachers can be very prone to this, as can store staff working under hot lights. Days off or holidays never seem to give trouble and are therefore great clues.

4. Is the first morning sample dark and stinging? Look closely at your previous evening's liquid intake and social activities. Perhaps you drank a lot and got up a few times in the night? By 7.30 a.m. there may be nothing left to pass. You must replace and rework the bladder function straight away, or a drying urethra may signal its unhappiness. Perhaps you didn't drink quite enough during the evening.

5. When you are off shift/duty/work, do you get twinges? Do they occur only at work? Do you drink regularly and void at work? If not, look to convenient points when you may instigate a change.

6. Coffee at work is all too common. Stop it for a week – you'll get withdrawal symptoms, probably headaches and irritability, but stick with it and see whether the twinges stop. If this works, allow yourself one weak coffee a day. Otherwise, a bottle of water in your desk will be a great help. No amount of workload or dutiful behaviour should cause ill-health. It is just not worth it.

If you do start a real attack of cystitis and you are pretty sure it is because of dehydration due to lack of liquid, you are best advised to follow the three-hour management programme on pages 15–16. Do everything as recommended, including the MSU sample (better safe than sorry!).

Cystitis caused by dehydration will respond very quickly to the management programme and clear up completely in the three hours. It may teach you a valuable lesson as well, because many women who have solved a previous problem with cystitis can get a bit blasé or careless. Women prone to cystitis occasionally need a lesson if they have let themselves down, and nothing pulls them up faster than another attack. It is a reminder from their kidneys, bladder and urethra that they require careful management – not risk-taking.

Antibiotics cannot help this kind of cystitis, nor will they do anything to counteract the dehydration. Antibiotics only work against an attack of cystitis caused by germs, nothing else. It isn't a good rule of prevention to rely on pills unless there is a background medical condition, such as the lack of oestrogen that comes with the menopause/a hysterectomy or old age. Then, of course, HRT in the form of pills of conventional or homoeopathic substances are very helpful, along with additional self-help measures, such as exercise.

Cystitis is a condition which is mainly self-imposed and mainly preventable by the patient. This understanding is the greatest advance since antibiotics stopped us from dying of it. Antibiotics don't stop attacks from starting, and that is where each patient's awareness, prevention and lifestyle make dramatic improvements over medical failure. Antibiotics can't work against non-bacterial causes – it is up to you!

Chapter 8

IRRITATION

Don't Scratch!

I suppose the first word associated with 'irritation', if you were asked, would be 'scratching'. If there's an irritation somewhere on your skin, it is natural to want to scratch it. But someone, often mother, always says 'Don't scratch, it will make it worse!'

We'll still try, perhaps with a gentle rubbing movement; and instantly the redness increases, the irritation increases. If it is scabrous, the scab can crack open and bleed; if it is dry, scaly skin, like dandruff or eczema, scratching isn't just with fingers – your whole body sets to in frantic motions and nothing else matters.

Usually, if you 'listen' to your body's vibes, it will tell you what it needs to help matters, like feeling thirsty makes you want to drink and reduces the dehydration balance. Not so, it seems, with irritation. Scratch at your peril!

If you scratch until you bleed, quite easily, the blood vessels become a railway for spreading the cause of irritation to other sites. All of us have done this at some time or other. My own worst times were during my cystitis years, 1966–1971, and a little beyond, when chronic vaginal thrush had broken out down my thighs and onto the labia, rooting deep in the hair follicles.

Heat from baths, bedding, underwear, trousers and simply the heat of my husband lying next to me were agonizing. In those years I woke us both during the night, scratching until blood ran quite freely. Scratching was unstoppable and getting up to dab with cold water in the bathroom was the only thing I could do to wrench myself out of it. It still didn't help much.

This scratching was so persistent that a patch of skin, deeply damaged by the combination of the scratching and the fungus, remained for years needing constant attention and calming creams. It did go finally. It is, of course, like twingeing or pain, a sign that something's wrong. Minor or major, something's not quite right and if it lingers we should do something about it.

Irritation anywhere along the perineum and inside the vagina, urethra, bladder or bowels brings additional difficulties. The most obvious ones are:

- It is too embarrassing to try to alleviate in front of anyone.
- No one can see it except yourself in the privacy of the bathroom.
- Much of it is internal, invisible and insufferable.
- Even walking round the house is uncomfortable.

There's another really important rule here for all women: *Don't put any old cream, ointment or antiseptic on it!*

Forget the adverts for 'intimate' creams; they are very deceptive and mostly worsen the situation either immediately or a few hours later. Only three things make any difference at all:

1. Finding the cause of the irritation as quickly as you can.
2. Resting – no walking.
3. Using a cool water bottle wash or even giving it a few minutes of the 'frozen pea bag' treatment. (Small size bag of frozen peas, wrapped in a clean cloth; don't ever eat the peas).

Causes

Until you are really aware of the specific cause for the particular irritation bothering you, any cream or pill is a matter of experiment and likely failure. Don't think the doctor is a fountain of knowledge guaranteeing diagnosis and treatment. The doctor is no better qualified than you, since only you feel the irritation. You must clearly explain and clearly show the symptoms.

On the couch, point to it if possible; tell when it started and whether you have experienced it before.

Bowel Irritation

Irritation of the bowels is often caused by foods or drinks. Irritation in the intestines, which lead into the bowel, can be due to either diarrhoea or constipation. Intestines can react within a couple of hours to a substance which they don't like. It is very individual, this allergy/sensitivity business. Most of us understand that cabbage, broccoli, peas and beans cause wind and bloating; not all of us double up with stomach pain when eating certain sorts of ice-cream or drinking filtered water!

The main allergy *groups* of *foods* are:

- cereals – wheat, barley, oats, corn
- pips and nuts – tomatoes, peanuts, pecans, grapes, etc.
- dairy products – milk, butter, yoghurt, cream, cheese, etc.
- pulses – lentils, peas, beans
- moulds – yeasts, fungi, cheeses
- spices, chemical additives – tartrazine, E types, hormones, many others
- fruits – citrus mostly – oranges, limes, grapefruits, lemons, citric acids, etc.
- shellfish – lobster, crab, prawns, oysters, mussels, etc.

Any or many can upset individual people.

'One man's meat is another man's poison' – which is where the great diagnostic difficulties for practitioner and patient begin. You are very lucky if the culprit becomes obvious quickly. An example of an easily traceable reaction might be vomiting after eating shellfish, or getting an immediate pain if you eat chocolate. Refined foods, like sugar, as compared with a natural honey, are often the worst and commonest causes of constipation. White flours and rice or other starchy foods come a close second, yet something like a curry can go straight through, perhaps even with a slight burning at the anal opening as it passes out.

Bowels excrete solid body wastes bound up by mucous and liquids which, unless bottle-washed off afterwards, remain suspended and travelling as a mixture up and down the perineum as we move. Any substances to which you personally have an allergy, together with their antibodies, can gain this additional external entry to the vagina and bladder. But first entry and reactions occur as the intestines sieve and sort valuable substances as against toxic, allergy-producing, unusable food particles. The liquids within foods (together with liquids proper) are also sorted, but are reserved in the bloodstream to be fully filtered by the kidneys. These will include toxic, unusable, allergy-causing particles in urine to be expelled, this time from the bladder.

Bladder Irritation

Bladder super-sensitivity can be ultra, ultra-sensitive in some women. Whether it is a diuretic substance or an infection/virus arriving via the bloodstream, the bladder will receive it and decide whether it is friend or foe.

Suppose you have such an irritating substance or liquid in your daily diet. It might have newly arrived because of a new change in your lifestyle. Perhaps you are a young mum and do the sandwich/cake routine now for children's teatime! Perhaps the new boyfriend smothers the candlelight dinners with black pepper! Perhaps it is winter and you are heavily into hot chocolate with cream! The list is endless for all ages and all situations. Just try to find what is different now from when you were well and did not have a sensitive, excitable bladder.

Finding the cause/s of your bladder trouble is a little easier if the increased frequency and pain from the bladder irritation is sporadic. Look back anywhere within the past 24 hours and see if you have eaten or drunk something slightly different. Maybe there is a favourite fish 'n' chip shop on the way home from your weekly Thursday hairdressing or business trip. Is it the same fish you choose each time, or could it be that the frying oil is nut-based (rather than vegetable-based) and nuts upset you? So Thursday night you make more trips to the bathroom and by Friday morning, the bladder nerve endings are well and truly signalling trouble.

It is impossible for a doctor, other than an allergy specialist, to begin sorting you out. Far better to have a go yourself first by observing your eating and drinking habits carefully.

When you think you might have an idea of the culprit, experiment with the food or drink and monitor your response. If the problem is continuous, look at the foods and drinks you eat on a regular basis, such as, for example, breakfast cereals, milk, fruit, chocolate, toast, cheese, mushrooms, jams, teas. Watch for any patterns, particularly if symptoms decrease at times or stop totally for a while. If you have to get up at night, what time was the last drink and what was it? I am still amazed at how many people have a coffee, chocolate or a similar hot drink at 10 p.m.! Obviously they're going to have to get up!

Vaginal Irritation

Not a lot of people, doctors included, know that allergic reactions can influence the vagina. Secondary bladder trouble caused by vaginal problems is discussed later more fully in Chapter 11, but is also worth a mention here.

Mucosal areas all over the body will secrete extra mucous if an allergic substance has entered your body. Noses run, eyes run, and vaginas can become more moist and itchy. Secretions, perhaps from too much fibre (particularly wheat bran) or from being pregnant, can and do cause vaginal mucous levels to rise. This leaks or drips out onto clothing. It also goes 'walk-about' up and down the perineum and can gain entry to the urethra.

Vaginal swabs show negative, the doctor doesn't know what else to do and the frustration is just too much on top of the symptoms. Too much fibre can cause all this extra leaking! Glandular activity and cell discarding increase (perhaps because of the fibre, perhaps as a result of another irritant), so more discharge forms. What to do?

The root questions if it is fibre are:

1. Why is so much fibre being taken?

   a) Because it is just a habit?
   b) Because bowels don't work unless it is taken?

2. Why are the bowels being stubborn?

   a) Because sugar intake is too much for your system?
   b) Because white flour and refined foods are clogging up the intestines?
   c) Because you take insufficient exercise?
   d) Because the wheat bran itself has clogged up the intestines?

e) Because you overeat?
f) Because of antibiotics or other medications?

Take any appropriate action on the above, then manage the drip:

- Remove the vaginal discharge and clean out the vagina morning and night.

Only after a full bottle wash (as described on page 65) may you then:

- Fill another 500-ml bottle with lukewarm water.
- Add to this a ¼-capful of Betadine solution, available at any pharmacy. Betadine is a great vaginal comforter.
- Pour this mixture very slowly down the perineum from the front (pelvic tilt position) – the procedure is carefully described on page 65 – don't change it!
- As the solution is running slowly down, insert the third/longest finger of your other hand up to the cervix and 'hook out' discharge from all round.
- Water and Betadine go inside as well, cleaning and clearing the vaginal walls of sticky, irritative mucous.
- Repeat five or six times until your finger exits clean of any trace of mucous.
- Dry carefully with a flannel – *not* towel or paper.

By cleaning out the vagina in the morning, dripping won't happen until early evening. Dripping only happens when the vagina can no longer hold the amount of discharge building up within itself. If the discharge is no longer dripping out of the vagina and onto your underwear, perineal and urethral soreness is not activated. Twingeing inside the urethra will calm down, especially if you increase your liquid intake for an hour or two to clean and calm the nerve responses. Pharmacies may want to sell you the Betadine kit with douche and gloves, but persist, if possible, on first buying the bottle of Betadine alone. It is an iodine-based liquid, but much distilled and diluted. Nevertheless, upset vaginas may not like it to begin with and it is often better to start cautiously with only a ¼-capful in the 500 ml of water. Increase to half a capful when you like and then a capful if required.

Understand that the vagina holds 24-hour influence over its neighbour, the urethral opening; that the urethral opening leads into the urethral tube and that this fine, short tube leads directly into the bladder. Only a sphincter valve, acting like a one-way gate, separates them, allowing urine its one-way downward flow. It does not prohibit a spreading of irritation or infection, so all adverse vaginal secretions setting up irritation at the urethral opening will certainly influence the urethral lining as well. Vaginal swabs are every bit as vital as urine samples for discovering the cause of cystitis; it is my feeling that both investigations should be done simultaneously. They seldom are.

I hope that you are beginning to understand how much the bowels and vagina influence the bladder. Keep these in good order and your bladder and urethra will be far healthier.

Thrush of the Bladder

Rather than repeat so many other publications on Thrush/Candidiasis/Monilia, I intend here merely to state the rules and give practical tips on avoidance and management.

Thrush breeds in alkalinity, moisture and warmth. Whether this is all provided internally or whether external factors (such as a hot bath or sweaty bedding) contribute, it matters not. Thrush eats sugar and yeasts, which certainly come primarily from food absorption, though this is also influenced by hormones, glands, enzymes and other bodily processes.

Thrush is always present in the gut, but upsurges when bacteroides (which break up foods) overgrow Bifidus bacteria (those tending to clean the intestinal lining). There is a constant battle between them and, so long as things are equal, there's no room for candida/thrush to get a hold. Once bacteroides gain ground, however, candida surges.

Understand that thrush of the bladder is a very real condition! It is much overlooked as a cause of cystitis and, sadly, most doctors don't accept it anyway. There is a urine test for it. Urine must be as highly concentrated as possible (preferably a sample taken when you first wake up). Microscopy should be done very quickly. These requirements can, as you may imagine, pose difficulties for NHS-run clinics/laboratories. Pay, if necessary, and plan the conditions carefully before taking the sample. Symptoms will be twingeing discomfort and ordinarily supervised urine samples may show up (wrongly) negative. The condition will worsen if you eat sugary foods or get hot. The appropriate medical treatment is Sporanox (an anti-fungal), for perhaps 10 days to two weeks if severe thrush or lengthy symptoms can be proved. Otherwise Sporanox is a seven-day course. Alternatively, a course of Diflucan is also helpful.

Thrush of the Gut and Bowels

It is in the gut that thrush begins. It is a fungus whose flagellae ('tails') hook onto the lining of the intestines and other sites to obtain nutrients for its reproduction and colonization. Eat sugar, chocolate, cream, yeast, fresh chunks of bread, mushrooms, alcohol, lots of fresh fruit, ice-creams, 'windy' foods, vinegars (French dressings, etc.), fruit juices, canned/bottled drinks or excessive carbohydrates such as flour, rice and pastas, and thrush will surge.

Symptoms in the gut may be bloating, wind, discomfort, gurgling, bleeding bowels. Haemorrhoids may swell and the anus may itch. Elsewhere on the body, the symptoms of a white tongue, sore throat, tiredness, lethargy, dark eyes exuding a whitish discharge, slightly blurred vision, a heavy head, ear exudation, vague tinnitus, dry mouth, tiny white spots on the gums and nasal blockage all can arise from a big gut upsurge.

From the gut upsurge, a general feeling of malaise can set in, contributed to in great part by many lifestyle conditions, such as:

- getting hot through exercise, hot weather, central heating
- being stressed, run-down, tired, slightly or seriously ill, working too hard
- soaking in the bath
- having sex when you or your partner are infected
- wearing tight clothing or nylon/polyester (anything that is not 100 per cent cotton) underwear
- drinking alcohol
- eating the wrong foods
- taking steroids for asthma or other illnesses
- taking antibiotics for any sort of illness; as the effect of antibiotics wanes only after three weeks
- taking anti-depressants long term
- having unbalanced hormone levels for whatever reason
- swimming in chlorinated pools
- having a viral illness such as ME (Myalgic Encephalomylitis) or HIV/AIDS
- being diabetic

Individual causes abound, one-offs that come to light only in counselling. Often there will be a cluster of small factors adding to a whole that culminates in upsurge.

Frequently the calendar can be responsible:

- Christmas/birthdays – alcohol
- Easter – finishing off all the chocolate eggs
- Summertime – lots of fresh strawberries/plums/peaches,

swimming, jam-making (and tasting!)
• Wintertime – layers of extra clothing causing sweating

It will be a waste of pills if taking them is the only treatment response. You, the patient, must reduce and remove whatever is at the source of the upsurge. Sporanox is strong and not to be taken any old time. Responsibility is shared again between patient, practitioner and pharmacy. Ignore this fact and the consequences will be continual trouble and frustration. Nystatin (sold as Mycostatin in the US and Australia) and Diflucan are all right as well, but Sporanox treats systemically – that is, it acts on candida present anywhere in the body, e.g. the sinuses, mouth, gut.

Thrush of the Vagina and Perineum

The vagina and perineum are secondary sites following the source in the gut. Symptoms, of course, are:

• an itchy, creamy, stringy discharge;
• red and swollen labia;
• itchy, swollen, reddened anus.
• acute phases can result in a heavy, purplish swelling of the labia with minimal or no discharge.
• walking can be painful and uncomfortable.
• haemorrhoids may swell and bleed

What to Do?

1. Get proof of the condition by (immediately) having a swab taken at the nearest genito-urinary clinic.
2. Eradicate all self-caused factors. I mean it! All of them!
3. Go to bed or take to your sofa in a long skirt, with no underwear, for as long as it takes.

4. Cut pubic hair to 1 in (2½ cm)
5. Cool-water bottle-wash the vagina three times a day.
   If vinegar in the bottle helps you, then add a capful to acidize vaginal mucous.
6. Take *only* three spoonfuls of a Bifidus-added plain live yoghurt before meals.
7. Increase liquid intake to prevent thrush rising into the urethra.
8. Don't walk, exercise or have sex.
9. Take oral anti-fungal medication (e.g. Sporanox) *and* a course of pessaries.
10. Insert the pessary *at night*, once you are in bed – and don't move afterwards!
11. The pessary *must* be pressed up against the cervix, not lower. Wear a sanitary towel.
12. Do you still need the steroids or antibiotics? Assessment is important.

Sexual Non-bacterial Irritation and Bruising

Diagnosis
Apart from urine samples being well and truly negative, not even showing any plus signs (++) in the cell, pus, blood or protein boxes, nor any influence from a recent course of antibiotics or prior 'comfort' drinking, there remains another accurate way of helping to diagnose bladder irritation or bruising caused by intercourse as against true urinary infection.

Timing
Germs take 24 to 48 hours to exhibit symptoms, though I have seen very exceptional circumstances, such as the woman whose bacterial cystitis began 12 hours after sex, and the woman who

did not present symptoms until 50 hours afterwards.

The 12-hour case was the result of using a bidet after diarrhoea and just before she was penetrated; in the 50-hour case a little (though ineffective) hygiene had been attempted. In the first case there was a heavy presence of coliform to start with; in the second case the presence was so low that it could only barely manage to stay active. But manage it did, with the 'help' of time, sex and an incomplete hygiene routine.

Mostly, sexually-activated bacterial cystitis will commence symptoms of an attack somewhere between 24 and 48 later, without any intermediate signals at all.

In the case of non-bacterial irritation or bruising, however, soreness, swelling and inflammation can commence even during sex, building within hours to an attack, still without bacteria.

These signs of soreness disturb the urethral and bladder nerve endings during intercourse. They get 'excited', 'stimulated', 'upset' and react by telling you that urine needs to be passed. Minutes later, they repeat the demand, and then again and again.

What to Do?

Drink half a pint (10 fl. oz/250 ml) of water immediately and take three strong painkillers to block the 'excitement'/'stimulus'. Clean and calm the vagina with a lukewarm bottle wash and place a comforting hot-water bottle at your back. Drink a glass of water or mild tea every 20 minutes until the bladder feels calmer or urine stops burning, or even do the three-hour management routine (see pages 15-16). Forget the sex!

What Could Have Caused It?

Full documentation of individual causes here is impossible. The circumstances of each woman's and each man's lovemaking are, of course, highly individual. All I can do is to give ideas and a few examples, to help you help yourself find the answer to your own problem.

TIMING.
Look again at the timing:

Does your soreness or 'reaction' start before sex?
Can this be related to the contraceptive you are using? Could it be a pessary, a cream, a contraceptive foam, a contraceptive sponge, the lubricant on a female condom, perfume sprayed accidentally onto the inner labia when only a dab on each inner thigh was intended, uninformed and incorrect use of any soap on the vulva (vaginal/urethral openings); a hot bath rather than the recommended bottle washing procedure; a hot bubble bath; a swim or a session in the jacuzzi; a vaginal infection that you are pretending isn't there; depilatory cream on pubic hair; wrong use of an antiseptic or deodorant to disguise a strong odour; dry menopausal skin; sitting on a jean seam in the car all afternoon so the vulva is already restricted and bruised?

All of these, and probably many more, are set up by you, the owner of the poor vagina about to be further mistreated. No doctor is going to fathom out this sort of cause! You've got to!

Does your soreness or 'reaction' (or even pain) start during sex?
I take an understanding of '*during sex*' to be any time from the first moment of foreplay of any sort, right through the duration of all sex acts, to stopping all genital/digital contact.

Again, can this be related to contraception? Often we stop quickly to insert or to put on barrier contraceptives. Does this cause an instant reaction? When the vagina is already warming up and blood vessels dilating, they may be more sensitive to creams and lubricants.

Oral/genital/hand contacts are minefields of prospective soreness. Think about beards, moustaches, 'designer stubble', strong tonguing, broken nails, dirty hands, insensitive finger work, one-spot only massaging, dildos, cucumbers, exotic condoms – you know the answer, no one else!

SIZE

Yes, he can be too big and too hard! Either let him ejaculate early (inside or out), or give him up! Once the early ejaculation has decreased the hardness, try him again. Use a good lubricant jelly, not Vaseline or spittle or anything else you feel like trying. Use a slow, gentle entry. Don't let him push and shove if it is hurting; try less penetrative positions and always change positions. Vaginas and bladders don't appreciate being pummelled in one place for half an hour (or longer!). If you sit on top, take control. Just one thrust up from him when you are pushing down is an earth/moon collision, with cervical bruising a real possibility.

Any tearing of vaginal skin internally or at the entrance may split and bleed. You wouldn't rub a cut finger, so change position and protect the vagina, or else stop. Lubrication with *KY Jelly* and slow entry do reduce this problem significantly.

Surprisingly, short sex sessions, where pent-up emotions are a driving force and niceties are ignored, can traumatize and bruise more than sessions where slowness and gentleness over an hour might have appeared more likely to cause trouble.

Sex between real lovers isn't just genital; it is stroking, caressing, licking, talking, appreciating the music, communicating, experimenting.

Does your soreness or irritation start after sex?

All sorts of sex – bar violence or rape – are quite OK so long as real soreness or bruising do not occur. Every woman 'feels' the intercourse afterwards – a bit swollen and sensitive – it can be lovely in its way. Steps to calm it all down are easy and helpful.

Cool Water Bottle Washing Procedure (for after sex)

- Go to a *warm* bathroom!
- Wash hands and fill one or two 500-ml bottles with coolish water, not hot.
- Sit on the lavatory and pass urine.
- Now do the pelvic tilt (backbone downwards).
- From the front, slowly pour the tepid water down the perineum and clean off sexual secretions.
- Insert the longest finger of your other hand and reach to the cervix, 'hooking out' more secretions, five or six times in and out as the water is trickling, so that this coolness cleans and calms the vagina. Use a second bottle, if needed.
- Stand up and pat dry with the flannel kept for perineal drying.
- Rest now! At least 10 minutes with your feet up and no underwear! Best of all, go to bed for a night's sleep. Drink a glass of water before you go.
- If it has simply been a heavy sex session, you will still benefit from the above cool water vaginal cleansing. Wash again in the morning. If your contraception prevents this, just wash down the outside.

Once all sexual activity has ceased, nothing more can actually cause soreness, bruising or irritation unless you stupidly take a hot bath, pull on a pair of jeans, go riding or even do a three-mile walk. The simple but incredibly effective cool water bottle wash stops all trouble.

Summary
So, sexually:

- A full bottle wash within six hours before sex cleans germs off and prepares the perineum. You can do a vaginal bottle wash as well if it is a bit 'stale'.
- Passing urine, using the cool water vaginal bottle wash, resting and drinking prevents soreness/bruising after sex.

All of which leads to lots of happy, cystitis-free sex! Take my word for it!

Menopausal/Advanced Age/Hysterectomy Irritation

Women coming to me who fall into one or more of these categories usually use the words 'deep irritation', 'dull pain', 'constant twingeing', 'dragging' or 'soreness' to describe their symptoms. They pinpoint external and/or internal sources of their discomfort.

Additionally, they may complain of aching wrists, neck and knees; tiredness, disturbed sleep; attacks of either bacterial or non-bacterial cystitis that only commenced with the menopause/after their hysterectomy; hot flushes; loss of libido; sweats and, of course, irregular periods (if they are still having them at all).

Hormone Replacement Therapy (HRT), if appropriate, can alleviate or lessen all these symptoms, not just the irritation and cystitis. If the first HRT prescribed isn't quite right, there are many more. There are also different ways of taking HRT:

- vaginal hormone creams
- oral tablets
- patches
- implants
- injections.

I suggest you read Wendy Cooper's books *No Change* and *Understanding Osteoporosis* (see Further Reading chapter for more information) for brilliant, comprehensive help, including a list of NHS/private clinics that offer HRT and of the differing hormone preparations. Mine is an oral tablet called Harmogen-oestrogen! Although it is American, it is available in

the UK on prescription (NHS or private) and very kind it is –
much kinder than Prempack or Premarin. Of course HRT is
not the answer for all women, nor is it always needed.

Bacterial Cystitis in Older Women
This is common to one-third of older women because a variety
of factors, including:

- stiff, arthritic joints preventing personal perineal washing
- ageing, atrophied perineal skin encouraging bacterial
  settlement
- diabetes or raised sugar levels causing thrush and urinary
  soreness
- urinary catheters
- dirty commodes in homes and hospitals

Environment

All environment these days is much dictated by fads and fash-
ions, all induced by our Western society. A consumer's gulli-
bility is again key. Bubble baths, for example, were not invented for health – they were invented for wealth – and not yours!
They irritate a woman's vulva if she is sensitive. Likewise soap
– it has got to be white, unperfumed and unmedicated for use
on the anus. Never, ever, soap the vulva (front part). Jeans literally bruise the urethral opening where the seams join. Loose
clothing prevents bruising, lets air circulate and protects the
body from potentially harmful chemicals.

Irritation in Babies, Little Girls and Teenagers

Bacterial Irritation

Bacterial attacks in youngsters are again caused entirely by an absence of hygiene or by ineffective hygiene procedures. Bottle washing is inappropriate for small children, but one bath a day should be quite adequate. If it can be done after she has passed a stool, fine. If not, then the daily bath will be important. Soap her back passage thoroughly as she stands up for you, then sit her down and make sure all the soap goes and isn't trapped. Don't soap her vulva – it may sting and it isn't necessary anyway.

Non-bacterial Irritation

Children don't know anything about hygiene. What mother and father impose upon them is for better or worse. All the little routines, foods, drinks, soaps and timings are fraught with possible trouble-spots leading to sore bottoms. Irritation and soreness followed by pain when they urinate is heartbreaking to watch. Somewhere in the child's daily life, either at home, at playgroup or at school, lies the cause. Neglecting to investigate and remove the cause will condemn the child to great unhappiness, lasting drugs, frightening hospital treatments, disrupted sex later on and maybe kidney infection and permanent scarring.

Even without bacteria, rising inflammation still causes the same distress, especially when scarring begins in earnest. Urethra, bladder and kidneys all bear scarring permanently whether it is caused by severe inflammation, infections or surgery. Parental awareness and the playgroup/school situation need sorting out before the child can be sorted out.

Foods and Drinks

Everything I have written about adult food and drink reactions applies to children. Allergies are often inherited and the new discovery of a gene that can predispose a person to asthma or allergies will throw light on these problems as research continues. For now it is a matter of accepting that, either in the same form or slightly different ones, a child can also show signs of allergic reactions.

Check List

- No fruit juices.
- No sugar-laden canned, cartonned or bottled drinks – except as a treat.
- No sugar-laden foods.
- Limit fruit intake to one piece a day.
- Make sure she passes urine at reasonable intervals at home and school.
- Make sure she drinks enough at reasonable intervals at home and school.
- Change underwear each day.
- No bubble baths or antiseptics in the bath.
- Use only a plain white soap for anal cleaning, none on the vulva.
- No antiseptics or creams on genital skin.
- Beware soreness after swimming in strongly chlorinated pools.
- Make sure she wears cotton knickers and skirts, dresses or loose trousers – *never* jeans.
- Teach her to clean herself properly after a bowel movement – wiping with toilet paper from behind and not touching the front.
- Check out the washing powder/liquid used in laundering – biological brands in particular can cause irritation.

These are the main guidelines, highlighting the commonest causes of childhood genital irritation and soreness. Take note!

When your daughter falls in love and wants sex, it may be down to you if she can't because of urethral damage. Strong words – I make no apologies!

A Couple of Other Triggers

Cold

Windy bus stops, gardening in a stiff breeze, sitting on a stone wall, all seem to affect some women, particularly older ones. It is not bacterial, it is irritation caused by dehydration. The cold stimulus upon kidneys and bladder sets the 'excitor' process off. Urine is passed several times, each successively more concentrated. Replacing this excreted liquid with a couple of warm drinks straight away – maybe even a bath or certainly a warm-up somewhere cosy – should redress the balance and comfort the bladder's 'excited', irritated nerve endings.

Car Travel

This can be a source of trouble, especially in older, less well-sprung cars on long journeys over bad roads. Again, many older women seem to cite this as, in the past, causing their irritation. Perhaps in truth they had a latent, undiagnosed bladder problem. In any case, with the advent of better cars and better roads I believe this sort of irritation to be on the wane. If it is a bother, then take along a good pillow to sit on, change your car, travel by train, and/or try painkillers to ease the bladder's nerve endings a little.

Chapter 9
CHEMICAL CONTAMINATION

Practically anything coming in contact with genital skin is man-made. I can hardly name a product that has not been dyed, coloured, treated or added to in some way, which tempts us from the supermarket shelf. Obviously, Rule 1 is: go for the simplest, least colourful, least added-to products you can find.

The Usual Suspects

Soaps

Only use white, unperfumed, unmedicated, undeodorized soaps. Shower gels, salts, bubble baths, medicated wipes, antiseptic soaps, deodorized soaps and more are packed with chemicals. I have heard *Knights Castile*, *Camay*, *Wrights Coal Tar*, *Cidal*, *Palmolive* and *Fresh* all cited as trouble-makers of genital soreness by sensitive women. Again, always go for the simplest sort and remember never to soap the urethral and vaginal openings. These areas of the body are not greasy and will not have a great colony of bacteria like the anal opening, which certainly has to be cleaned with a soapy hand, as described in the full bottle washing procedure on page 65.

Deodorants

Never deodorize the vulva or anus; wash them properly with bottle washing. Do not use deodorized tampons.

How to Reduce Vaginal Odour

- Bottle wash daily as described.
- Then do a vaginal bottle wash; add the Betadine, occasionally, if necessary (see page 101).
- Keep pubic hair cut to 1 in/2½ cm in length to avoid the retention of odours and fungi.
- Wear cotton underwear.
- Keep the perineum comfortably cool.

Antiseptics

Most antiseptics sting and irritate. Never use them on the perineum. Proper bottle washing removes any need for them. Do not use pure antiseptic for bathroom cleaning, especially never on the loo seat. Always remove all trace of cleaning fluids with a carefully rinsed cloth, and prevent any splashing up from the pan water when you pass a stool by placing one sheet of toilet paper on the water's surface beforehand.

Shampoos and Shower Gels

Would you have spotted these as the possible cause of irri-

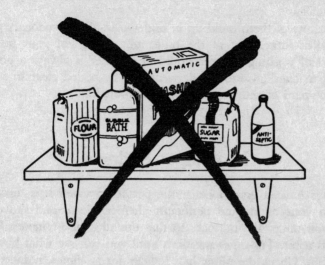

tation? A man or woman using them can risk chemical contamination of the penis or vagina. This might then be transmitted as an irritant during intercourse. Shampoo used on little girls' hair, in the bath because this is convenient and easy, may immediately or over time transmit irritant chemicals via the rinsing and the bath water to her sensitive vulva. Worst for this are the antiseptic sort and any containing hexachlorophene. Symptoms might start immediately with a new bottle or might build up over several weeks of bath times using a variety of shampoos.

Bubble Baths

Ghastly! A major cause of non-bacterial irritation, soreness, discharge, urethral stinging and cystitis. Use them, buy them at your peril. They should carry a government health warning. I mean it!

Washing Powders/Liquids and Fabric Softeners

All or any of them build up in underwear. If you suddenly get a cystitis attack out of the blue, any change of your usual brand of washing powder/liquid or softener is always a good thing to check. Cotton underwear can be boiled clear in successive pans of water to remove contamination.

Looking at Redness

Always have a good look at the perineum when it is 'upset'. Wash your hands and perineum, then lie down and shove a cushion under the buttocks so that this tilts the perineum forwards a bit. Try other positions until you can see what has to be seen. Check the pubic hair follicles for swellings, redness or itchiness. Then part the fleshy outer labia and, holding a magnifying mirror, move your fingers around, feeling and looking for the site and possible source of the trouble.

Examine any scars – such as those left by an episiotomy or tears – feel for any bumps, lumps or spots; check whether the anus is red and oozing, likewise the vaginal opening. Ring a special clinic if the perineum needs swabbing and professional examination.

Do not clean out the vagina before going for swabs and do not drink too much so that a urine sample becomes diluted.

Chapter 10

CLOTHING

A Brief History of Underwear

Only since the 1940s have women worn close-fitting knickers. Cotton, or silk if you were rich, were natural, breathing materials, soft enough for women to wear next to their skin. In the 1920s and 1930s, the French cami-knicker in silk, voile or very fine cotton lawn was loose with a crotch low enough not to get caught up between labia or buttocks when sitting. Before that, Edwardian women wore longer pantaloons/bloomers secured at the waist with tie-strings and at the knees with pretty ribbons, all very loosely crotched and of cotton.

Victorian women wore these too, but because the crinoline gowns made bathroom/garden privy visits a near impossibility, they had wide open crotches which were very much easier for squatting on potties. Potties were positioned all over the home – in bedrooms, naturally, but also anterooms and small 'retiring rooms' which afforded a little privacy. The same sort of underclothes and petticoats were worn by all classes and each home had several potties.

Beyond Victorian times open crotches were absolutely normal for underwear. Layers of petticoats and the long pantaloons were women's standard clothing, necessary for coping with life in cold, unheated homes. Open-crotched underwear and petticoats were seldom removed even in bed, so sexual access was also provided for.

What a long way we have 'progressed'! Modestly and alluringly, we cover up our perineum in gusseted, closed styles of underwear. We use cotton in all weights and colours and we use nylon/viscose/rayon to create patterned or see-through glimpses of flesh. Gussets of man-made materials, even those with a cotton inner lining, are non-porous, air-inhibiting garments.

We may prefer a seamless gusset for comfort and we certainly no longer have the extended protection of long cotton petticoats, but do we have to wear this underwear all the time? Do we really have to deny our perineums the air which their naturally open physiology requires?

We have very moist perineums and normal discharges. If we add on sweat or perspiration to the moisture, we greatly encourage the spread of bacteria and fungus infestation. Think of the foot and toe fungal problems that have arisen since the advent of trainers and other types of running shoes. Think of the upsurges of thrush and dermatitis since tights, leotards and leggings arrived.

I would lay money on these fungi as being modern, not much encountered before the 1940s and hardly at all before the 20th century. Be user-friendly and remove your underwear when you are at home. Only buy 100 per cent cotton knickers, without that biting seam which some manufacturers sew on the crotch joins. Keep an air flow around your perineum at all times.

This then being the rule, if you want to stay genitally/sexually healthy, take a look at the clothes you wear for business, sports and hobbies to see how, in these unavoidable situations, you can still treat the perineum properly.

At Home/Work

Home Clothes

- Keep warm with long body vests/T-shirts, slips/petticoats.
- Keep cool with longer cotton dresses in the summertime.
- Wear culottes or longer woollen skirts rather than trousers.
- Go without leotards.
- Go without underwear when convenient and comfortable.
- Wear cotton knickers.

Work Clothes

- Wear cotton knickers.
- Don't wear unbreathing tights which create moisture.
- Don't wear trousers; wear culottes in any natural cloth according to the season if your job requires this sort of clothing.
- Check the office chair: Is it propelling your knickers for six hours at a time up into the sensitive vulval skin? Shift your position every so often; take a soft feather cushion to sit on. Walk around frequently to aerate the perineum.

Sports Activities

Swimming

Choose a clear water pool, not cloudy from chlorine; peer closely at its contents – any stringy, jelly-type substances floating about? Don't touch it! Likewise, if it is green, slimy and heavily used – don't go near it. I've had two pools closed in my time and I've caught *Gardnerella* in a famous private members' pool! Trust nothing – examine it. If it seems OK, then swim, jacuzzi sensibly (for no more than seven minutes) and get out. Then:

- shower straight away
- dress
- go to the cloakroom, fill the 500-ml bottle in your bag, pass urine and then bottle wash the vagina and perineum to remove most of the chemicals found in pool water.

Sea-bathing can give you brain damage these days! Even if it is a quiet bay somewhere, check with locals that it isn't quiet because they all know the sewage outlet is there! Check out factory waste and all the other relevant environmental factors (the media is usually quite good at keeping us up to date on any hazards). Back at the guest house, clean out the vagina just to be on the safe side!

Obviously, you have no choice but to wear a swimsuit. Rinse it thoroughly and change rather than let it dry on you. You may notice other women standing at the pool-side shower, their backs to you, fiddling away down the front of their swimsuit to clean the vulva! Quite right, too!

Keep Fit, Aerobics, Work-outs, Gyms

This is all about sweating! Elevated body temperatures give candida/thrush the green light for upsurging. Thrush loves heat and usually where there is heat, there is sweat. Pubic hair perspiration helps fungus embed itself in and between hair follicles. Even if attempts are made to cool down, the combination of non-porous leotard crotches, several leotards worn together, the exercise heat and the amount of time spent exercising will all conspire to lengthen the time spent sweating. Even after a shower it can still be some time before you cool down and stop sweating entirely.

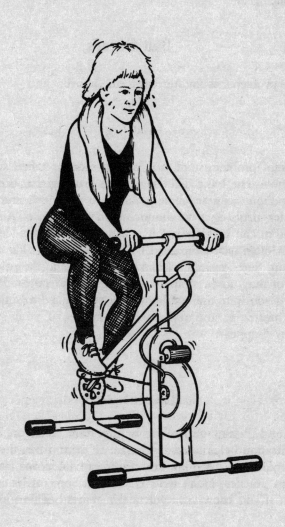

I find that sick women will have stopped exercising because they just cannot manage it anymore, but some struggle on, further depleting their lowered immune system. I advise cystitis/thrush patients not to exercise until they are perfectly well again.

Ball Games

Same problems as for Aerobics, etc., above.

Riding

Different problems, unless it is high summer when sweating is common. The basic difference is the bruising that occurs: from the jodhpur/jean seam pounding into the vulva and a higher bladder bruising from bouncing in the saddle. An unusual symptom can be bleeding. It is blood from the bladder/urethra and is often *un*accompanied by other symptoms like frequency or pain. Soreness and a feeling of heaviness in the pelvic region may or may not accompany spotting on underwear. Play detective: If you were fine until you took up riding – or any sport for that matter – stop for a while and see if your symptoms lessen/disappear.

Laundering

Obviously, clean underwear is important. Bacterial or fungal colonization in dripped discharge or urine from the previous day makes wearing knickers for more than one day a hazardous practice. Don't wear knickers in bed – air is essential at night. If you know your vulval skin reacts badly to all washing powders/liquids, then choose dark-coloured cotton underwear and boil it clean. This may mean frequent shopping for new pairs, because only washing powders/liquids remove the stains.

If such sensitivity is not a problem, then just wash your underwear along with the rest of your normal load. Machines rinse pretty well these days, but you could always give your underwear an extra hand rinse if desired.

Chapter 11
LIFESTYLE

In this one word, lifestyle, lies 80 per cent of the reasons for both sorts of cystitis – bacterial and non-bacterial. Everything written in this book so far supports this.

Lifestyle factors can never be stressed strongly enough. No patient, doctor (or nurse or other health professional) can ever spend too much time discussing the events, patterns or habits of the sufferer's life and her home, work and leisure-time pursuits.

Until I began my work in 1971, a patient's involvement with her own cystitis was absolutely nil.

'Take the pills; take more of the pills; take the pills indefinitely!'

'It is a part of woman's lot!'

'You need tranquillizers, you're imagining it!'

'Have a baby, that works sometimes!'

'We'll dilate the urethra again!'

'You're hysterical!'

Frustration was enormous for patients and doctors; textbooks were impractical and unreadable. No literature existed to redress the medical lethargy and ignorance and to begin to place the power and control firmly in the hands of the patient.

The first light at the end of the tunnel was the three-hour

management procedure and the realization that passing water after intercourse helped. Suddenly the concept of a woman doing things at home to help herself began to gain credence. Neither myself nor anyone else involved with cystitis research has ever looked back to the bad old days. All around the UK (and other countries), hospitals, surgeries, nurses, teaching departments, magazines, TV and radio and countless ex-victims are providing more and more testimonials to the success of self-help methods for fighting cystitis.

Principles

All the major principles of self-help are now in place. Each new sufferer must simply get acquainted with them as quickly as possible. Cystitis will always exist, and will always erupt in those sensitive to it. Helplines, leaflets, programmes, books, videos and telling and helping others are the ways in which we can all gain and give advice about what to do – without having to go to the doctor each time for pills.

One morning my phone rang at 9 a.m.; the woman who had rung was coping with her first ever attack (which had begun at 4.30 that morning!). It was the soonest I had ever been brought in to advise on an attack (the previous record had been three weeks, again after a first bout).

In the early years of my work, when material was not widely available and suffering was terrible, I ran a 24-hour help line; nowadays I get a bit annoyed if I am rung out of office hours, because so much other help is available. Friends can help you; the book shop or library; the doctor's surgery; the pharmacy – so many sources of help are at hand. Of course, if any woman has read and deliberated over this book and still needs counselling I will offer it, but the message is to help yourself, using all the carefully researched and described principles laid out here. Don't think you know better than me and change basics. If I say a 500-ml bottle, I truly mean it; others have been tried and have failed for specific reasons; if I say that three to five pints (60–100 fl. oz/1½–2½) of liquid a day should be drunk, I mean it. Ignore, change or bend the rules and you will find out that I was right. Read, absorb and digest slowly and carefully.

Having said all this, I teach the principles and give plenty of additional help by examples. What I cannot be expected to account for are the thousands of habits and circumstances that 25 million UK households practise.

Last autumn I lectured at a large hospital, from which a doctor referred a 'very difficult' patient to me in London. I can't tell the whole story, which included incorrectly taken urine samples that gave false results, job stress, HRT and a high sugar intake, but I will tell you of just one exchange I had with this woman:

'And you've bottle-washed after passing a stool, as I advised?'

'Absolutely, yes.'

'How often do your bowels open? Every day, every other day?'

'Oh, no! Every 13 days and it just seems to explode!'

No one, except someone with a severe bowel adhesion, goes that long and lives! Yet despite all the pills, liquids, etc., this had been her lot. What caused it? I found she'd had a severe addiction to sugar since childhood. Desperate, and now in her late thirties, she stopped sugar on my suggestion and – hey presto! – her bowels now happily open without any help, every other day. My advice was: bottle wash after passing a stool without fail. I would never have thought to account for a *13-day interval* between bowel movements! No wonder things still weren't right!

Patient's Approach

The only acceptable changes in bottle washing, for instance, may be in patients who have disabilities such as Multiple Sclerosis, arthritis, paraplegia or the many other diseases or injuries that make one's movement or strength uncertain. But these changes should and can be designed to suit each individual.

I won't accept laziness or sloppiness when health is at stake. I like a patient who tries; if she is not quite sure about something, I will help to correct it. I won't accept sheer stupidity though:

'Well, why aren't you doing the bottle washing after every bowel movement?'

'Because it makes such a mess.'

'No it doesn't. How are you making it make a mess?'

'Well, you demonstrated it to me with your clothes in place. I always have to pull my skirts up and pull my knickers down when I'm on the toilet. I just can't do it like you!'

Of course I keep my clothes on for demonstrations! I'm not undressing in front of other people. *Of course*, if it is for real, in my bathroom, I pull my knickers down and hold my skirt up, like everyone else!

I hate cystitis on my own behalf and on all other victims' behalf, but my sympathy is limited. What is required is hard attacking, individual diagnosis, and resulting actions. It is a battleground and I have come from the ranks to be the Commander. I fight and control, so must you.

Gynaecological Problems

These can include the gynaecologist! He or she may be disastrous, not spotting the problem in the first place, adding to the problem, or causing an additional problem.

I saw a woman last year who took away with her a long list of ideas and suggestions. Nine months later she rang and, though her symptoms had improved, they had not gone entirely. We ran through my list and she had complied with everything except the first suggestion – to see a gynaecologist in London since her local ones had not found anything wrong. My hunches tend to be accurate. Persuaded, she came down to London and, within 40 minutes of seeing a gynaecologist there, a growth, now the size of a plum, had been discovered in the cervical canal. Urgent phone calls followed and she was admitted to hospital in her area, London being too distant. She is now improving.

Doctors are human, yet we put an abnormal amount of trust in them. Just because they have passed exams does not mean they are all-knowing. Always get a second opinion, and even question test results closely. Practically every gynaecological problem can affect the bladder and urethra, which, after all, lie in close proximity to the uterus and vagina. There are many ways in which our reproductive organs can cause trouble in the bladder and urethra.

Retention of Urine before a period and causing cystitis, stinging, bloating or thrush is probably a matter of hormones. See to these and symptoms decline. For some the problems may be resolved by taking the contraceptive Pill; for others Evening Primrose Oil, close attention to diet and exercise, and a daily diuretic pill from the pharmacy or doctor during the week before a period may help. *Aci-Jel* vaginal jelly inserted at night for a week balances the alkalinity which arrives before a period and which helps thrush breed faster if it is present.

Pregnancy may bring on or stop cystitis and/or urinary frequency. The cause may be the heavier vaginal discharge that accompanies pregnancy and can irritate the urethra, or haemorrhoids, which can cause cystitis by harbouring faecal bacteria in their crevices. Weight from the baby and from hormonal change can bring on frequency.

Rest up when possible. Do a vaginal bottle wash morning and night to clear out the discharge regularly. A full bottle wash after a bowel movement cleans off the residue on haemorrhoids.

Childbirth can lead to cystitis (either bacterial or non-bacterial) while you are in hospital. Bacterial cystitis can come from catheterization, tearing, stitching or dirty commodes, bidets and lavatory seats stained with blood and debris. Line the seat with toilet paper before using it. Carefully wash your perineum before actual delivery, if possible. Bottle wash daily in hospital to keep external stitching clean. Dry carefully and expose the perineum to plenty of air. Place pads underneath and let the vulva be exposed beneath your nightie or sheet.

Non-bacterial cystitis is usually caused by bruising during the baby's emergence. Rest, coolness and painkillers will all help after a few days. Any antiseptics known to cause cystitis must be avoided. Be firm: 'Don't swab me with any sort of antiseptic please. I have washed very carefully and antiseptics give me cystitis!'

Haemorrhoids and episiotomy scars are a common cause of cystitis after childbirth. Only daily bottle washing stops faecal germs harbouring or travelling to the urethral and vaginal openings.

Menopause/Hysterectomy often cause soreness, dryness, cystitis, stinging. Lowering hormone levels do not just make our faces wrinkle. They also make our urethras, vaginas and perineums wrinkle. It is called ageing, or atrophy. Skin gets thin, cracks and encourages bacterial growth. Sex is dry and miserable. Local creams, oral treatment, patches or implants will restore urethral, vaginal, perineal, sexual and bladder health.

Old Age is a major cause of cystitis. It is hormonal. Stiffening wrists, arms or necks prevent easy perineal cleaning. Commodes need daily cleaning and all the factors mentioned for the menopause apply, but even more so. Catheters and pads can cause soreness, bleeding and infection. Hormones can definitely be prescribed to older women. Doctors are happy now to prescribe them for 40-, 50- and 60-year-old women, but have not quite understood that they can help 70- and 80-year-olds! Keep pushing! If you are choosing a nursing home, ask to see the bathrooms, lavatories and kitchen – never mind the lounge!

Ovarian Cysts if left untreated may cause symptoms throughout the reproductive organs and influence the urethra, causing stinging and frequency. Another sign of cysts may be a stiff back.

Polyps anywhere in the uterus, cervix or vagina can cause secondary stinging and cystitis. Polyps usually ooze and retain organisms which become a drippy discharge and affect the vulva and urethra.

Vaginal Thrush can and does cause perineal soreness, irritation, urethral and bladder pain and also cystitis. If it is cyclical, use Aci-Jel vaginal jelly to increase vaginal acidity (which declines before a period). If it is present at other times, check:

- your sexual partner – is he a beer/alcohol drinker, a heavy sugar/cheese eater?
- your diet – do you eat a lot of cheese, cream, sugars, yeasts, chocolate, mushrooms, 'windy' foods, *excessive* bread/rice/potatoes? Do you drink a lot of alcohol or canned/cartonned drinks?
- your bedding – nylon, dacron, terylene duvets, nylon nighties or panties? Remember too, to keep cool – use cotton or

other natural fibres wherever possible.
- your job – too hard, too energetic? Your work clothes too constricting/non-cotton? Are you sitting all the time? Is your energy depleted?
- illness – ME (viral fatigue), flu, HIV/AIDS, cancer and many other serious illnesses, or just being tired and run-down, can all contribute to thrush.
- drugs – antibiotics, steroids, ulcer drugs, antacids?
- your hobbies – elevated body temperatures, leotards, swimming?
- your clothing – nylon underwear, tight skirts, jeans, leggings, corsets?

Remember:

- Keep cool; avoid sugar, certain drugs, certain clothes, men (for a while, anyway!); change jobs if you can, monitor your hobbies.
- Keep well and fresh, take oral and local anti-fungal treatments when you are hit by a big upsurge of thrush.

Erosions of the cervix can cause soreness, frequency and/or cystitis. Symptoms like these and an exuding erosion require that it be removed. Symptoms will then cease. You might have to fight for this.

All Vaginal Infections can cause secondary non-bacterial cystitis. Inflammation from chlamydia, gardnerella, trichomonas and lots of other bacteria or parasites spreads out and on to the perineum. Urethral contact is quickly established and the sensitive nerves begin to react. Only a vaginal swab will disclose the specific vaginal infection and then the correctly sensitive antibiotic. Urinary symptoms will correspondingly decrease. Don't bottle wash for 12 to 15 hours before the swab is taken or the swab result will be negative.

Herpes can cause urinary stinging during an outbreak or even full-blown (non-bacterial) cystitis depending upon the site of the blisters. Read the literature on herpes and try to prevent it. Treat any outbreak instantly with one of the suggested medications. Lysine from any pharmacy – taken daily as a preventative, then more heavily if a blister appears – seems to be quite helpful in avoiding severe outbreaks. Stress levels from any source can activate this virus and its pain.

Thyroid/Endocrine Malfunctions can cause bladder pain. Other symptoms abound, but this book is about bladders. A really competent endocrinologist with many tests at his or her disposal can provide the best diagnostic and therapy results.

Surgery and Scarring negatively affect bladder and urethral tissue. Interference of any kind with nerve endings causes reactions such as twingeing, frequency, achiness and feelings of heaviness.

Of all pelvic organs, the exceptional sensitivities of the urethral and bladder nerve endings make reactions possible at any time. Careless scalpel work or bruising of the bladder during surgery can result in a lot of misery for the patient. Scar tissue may adhere, blocking or obstructing the bladder so that it cannot work to full capacity. Prolapse surgery needs great skill and care – not a quick hitch and a few ill-placed stitches. Dilatations scar forever and scar tissue decreases urethral and bladder function, even encouraging bacterial colonization in its weakened defences. In the United States surgeons have performed dilatations so frequently on cystitis sufferers that hundreds of thousands of women have been left with more scar tissue than natural urethral/bladder tissue. Inevitably, function is impaired and great pain ensures. Nor do dilatations stop infection from reoccurring.

Urological Conditions

Urinary Leaking/Incontinence.

There are many leaflets and much help available from continence advisers these days. They visit you at home to get a feel for your lifestyle and personal difficulties. They are fully trained nurses who have specialized in urinary care in order to help the huge numbers of women who suffer from leaking or varying degrees of incontinence. Ask at your doctor's surgery/local hospital for their help.

Leaking is more likely to occur in a woman who has experienced a difficult labour and has lost muscle tone on the perineum. The urethral sphincter valve (which lets urine out of the bladder) may also have stretched a bit, leaving a less tight seal when it is closed and the urethral opening may have distended a little also. There are good exercise books for strengthening the pelvic floor muscles but, once you get the hang of it, pulling up and tightening the perineum can be done sitting or standing with a minimum of fuss whenever you want.

If, as you get older, the problem of dribbling or leaking when you sneeze, laugh, bend down, etc. suddenly arises, ponder this: Skin, muscles, ligaments, organs, etc., etc. do lose tension and support over time. HRT (if appropriate) can help, but nature and ageing are inexorable. Slight weight gain (even as little as three pounds) can make the difference between the urethral sphincter managing to 'hold' urine within the bladder or being forced to allow a leak if sneezing, bending, etc., take it by surprise. Heavy weight gain poses greater problems: no ageing bladder or urethral sphincter can withstand a great downward pressure, and incontinence garments may have to be worn.

Keep the weight off, keep the bowels well moved, stay off sugars, fats, 'windy' foods, sweets, alcohol, etc. Exercise reasonably and tone up the perineum as often as possible. If the problem seems to be a prolapsed bladder, then get two opinions and good-quality scans. The uterus can sometimes by its own pressure relocate (prolapse) the bladder, in which case the uterus will have to be lifted away. Ask around among local nurses and among other women who may have had a prolapse operation, to assess whether one surgeon's operative success rate is better than another's! If you don't like a surgeon's attitude, don't trust his or her operative skills either. We have all had enough of 'You'll be all right, my dear, next patient please.' All doctors should have to take courses in counselling skills these days before they are given their degree.

Urinary leaking can also be a sign of a very low-grade bacterial infection of the urethra and bladder. This is common in older, arthritic women who don't shower, bath or wash as they need to. I know of women in their eighties who bottle-wash twice a day (morning and bedtime) without any difficulties. Implement this simple cleaning procedure, paying special attention to soaping thoroughly between and around haemorrhoids and then rinsing off from the front with the bottle until all the soapiness has dropped off down the loo. I lecture a lot to continence advisers and they swear by this routine. Disabled, injured, ill or incontinent patients have all stopped getting infections once the nurse has taught it to them or they have been shown my video.

I have said nothing about urological problems such as stones, diverticuli, reflux, stenosis and more. Usually one visit to a urologist and a scan, x-ray and cystocopy will reveal these sorts of problems. They are not everyday occurrences in general practice and because they are easily spotted early with urological diagnosis, such conditions never come my way.

Men

I have also neglected men. Obviously men get far less cystitis than women, but sexual infections can cause urethritis, or prostatitis in later years. Some homosexual acts and certain lifestyle causes such as heavy alcohol intake can also make for very miserable symptoms. Much in this book can also benefit any men who are in need of understanding and ideas.

In the Bathroom

Only three pieces of bathroom equipment are required for personal hygiene:

1. A lavatory
2. A basin
3. A bath/shower.

These are available absolutely everywhere. All homes from the humblest to the mightiest have these, so no excuses for smelling, please! Unfortunately, the perfect-shaped lavatory hasn't yet been invented. It ought to be an inch longer from seat front to seat back than it is at present, so that we would all have a little more room in front for bottle washing – but it is all quite manageable as it is. Bidets have many drawbacks:

- They cause vaginitis and cystitis.
- They aren't plumbed far enough away from the wall for leg room as you *face* the taps, so faecal germs run towards the vulva.
- Temperature control is impossible before water hits the vulva.

- Water doesn't travel upwards and round the corner to the anal opening, and if it does it will only run downwards to the vagina again with all the faecal germs.
- A central spray is a bacterial blender, not a clean front-to-back flow.
- It is a 'luxury' item and few homes have them, thank goodness!
- Hospital bidets are never to be touched! Filthy!

Washing Sequences

Separate lavatories create unnecessary difficulties for bottle washers because they must walk from the lavatory to the basin next door. There should be in every home at least one lavatory and sizable basin in the same room.

Showers are cheaper and better than baths (in terms of the spread of bacteria), but so long as bottle washing is the prime washing procedure, bathing twice a week (doing just the 'stand-up armpit-washing' routine on the other days) is acceptable; as is a shower every day – *after, not instead of* bottle washing. Please finish by facing the shower, parting your legs and checking by feel that no soap or shower gel is trapped on the perineum or between the labia to irritate the rest of the day or night.

A house move will involve differences in the new bathroom. Watch out for little things like the basin being so close to the lavatory that you think you won't have to stand up to soap the anus. You *do* still have to stand up! Body positioning and gravity are always important. Perhaps you have succumbed to the sparkling blue bidet and now there are vaginal swabs showing klebsiella on the cervix. Take the antibiotics and put a fern in the bidet!

Perhaps your cystitis starts every Sunday at your new

boyfriend's home? Does the central heating stay on so that bottle washing is done in a warm bathroom? Or is it too cold to get out of bed to do it?! Have you just bought a double bath for pre-sexual soaking – this is too hot, inflammatory and drying; sexual lubrication will be soaked away, though *KY Jelly* could remedy this. Does the lavatory get cleaned every day or does he share his house with some less-than-hygienic folk? Is the bathroom down the stairs and through the kitchen where everyone has congregated for a late evening supper and you don't feel like traipsing all the way in your nightie to run the gauntlet of winks and nudges?! No matter the hurdles, anything stopping you bottle washing when you should has to be corrected.

Changing
Homes/Boyfriends/Diet/Job/Exams

Homes

Stress! A house move, with all the cleaning, painting, drilling, gardening, entertaining – not to mention the money worries or discussions – this entails, can negatively affect anyone's hormones for a couple of months. Try a holiday – no money left? – try the well-woman clinic – cheaper! If it is not hormones it may be dehydration, irregular liquid intake when you actually need more at this time because of your increased physical activity. Perhaps you have taken to the bottle to celebrate or as an 'I *must* have a drink' comfort! Which rules have you bent, broken or neglected that kept cystitis at bay before?

Boyfriends

All sorts, extra-marital as well. Is the bathroom unsuitable? Are you bottle washing within six hours of sex? Does he insist that you have some wine too? Has a new need for contraception arisen? Does using this new sort coincide with the first sign of twingeing? Is he uncircumcised and not really cleaning the foreskin? Does he take you swimming, drinking, curry-eating, chilli-eating? Does he take you climbing, driving, diving? Anything to chafe, irritate, dehydrate? Does he have new (for you)/unusual sexual habits? What is his job – does he use chemicals, building materials, sit at a desk and have long nails? Check his underwear and towels too! The possibilities are endless and highly individual. Look to all these factors and more to find what has triggered your cystitis.

Diet

All sorts of social factors lead to dietary changes. Perhaps you have decided to become a vegetarian? Veggie foods cause bloating and farting, with the accompanying dangers of wind-borne expulsion of faecal germs. Have you gone to live abroad? Wherever it is, from New York to Adis Ababa, foods and liquids will be different enough to cause problems. Are diarrhoea or loose stools now a daily hazard? Maybe it is down to too much garlic in each meal, or drinking a different kind of tea. Perhaps you are suddenly eating more sugar, or are dehydrated, or comfort eating because of boredom. Look for the differences, experiment and then institute changes back to the old, safe ways. Constipated? Have you started eating meat or eggs every night? Are you favouring brewed coffee or pure orange juice nowadays for breakfast after that gourmet break in Bruges? Snacking on chocolate or fruit gums?!

Job

Who would think that daily work could influence the urethra and bladder!

First Question – did cystitis coincide with a career move, a change of office, a change of job, a change of boss, starting shift work?

Second Question – If so, how does this affect the primary causes of bacterial/non-bacterial cystitis (see below).

You may be able to pinpoint the exact date that symptoms began, or it may only be gradually that you become aware that 'something isn't right'. Once an idea forms, and proof of the problem borne out by a well-taken and accurate early morning urine sample – put the circumstances right and see if your symptoms decrease.

Is it Bacterial?

Do you now have to catch an earlier train, which means that instead of bowels opening before leaving, you have to wait until arriving at work? Bottle washing routines need careful, practical re-alignment (see Chapter 5).

Shift-work upsets some women's sensitive bodies. Be prepared to give it up if necessary – you may earn less but you will feel better. Did you forget to pack the bottle for a business trip? In its absence what was used – a mug? If so, there was probably not enough water to get rid of all the soap! Better to get a bottle from the bar – 500 ml or 2 x 300 ml. Try to think of *any possible* disturbance to your routine. It may be significant enough to have caused a bout of bacterial cystitis.

Is it Non-bacterial?

Is the new office chair pressuring the urethra from underneath and your weight pressing from above all day long? Blood vessels constrict, then expand, creating a slight swelling as they do so. Five days a week of this may mean a distinctly uncomfortable bladder by Friday night. Have the lads propelled you each lunchtime into the new wine bar for a quick drink – or two – or three on Fridays? Come 5 p.m. and dehydration may be causing twingeing. Drink mineral water, not alcohol. Is the person who cleans the cloakroom off sick? Always line the seat and sit comfortably. Is the boss too demanding upon your time/energy!?

Remember to drink and void at regular intervals.

Exams

Varying degrees of stress result in changes to our behaviour. 'Swatting' all day in the library in jeans/other uncomfortable clothing produces the same problems as office staff can encounter. Relaxing in the pub afterwards just adds insult to the day's inertia and lack of dietary care. Thrush may upsurge too, from the lack of air to perineal skin and too many chocolate bars for energy! Perhaps your underwear isn't being changed or washed properly and ageing mucous is starting to harbour bacteria, or maybe rinsing is less than satisfactory. If you are tired, thrush can upsurge and an early signal may be urethral twingeing. Pace yourself as best you can with regular meals and drinks, regular sleep, and a few hours to relax properly between study sessions.

Holidays

How many of us have had a much-needed, well-earned holiday ruined by cystitis or vaginitis of some sort?

The main thing is to step *up* the rules, *not* think, 'it'll be fine, I'm on holiday!' A holiday is a huge hazard, since too much of everything that can cause cystitis – sex, sun, swimming, heat/cold, alcohol, food, perhaps even stress – is the norm. Keep following all the rules, and have a great time. Keep a toothbrush in your bottle-wash bottle to stop the cleaners taking it away!

A Final Word

In the fight against cystitis, your efforts to self-diagnose (by taking a look at your lifestyle) are paramount. Reading this book and searching for clues are pre-requisites to success once urine sample results have accumulated and been understood. So much is caused unwittingly by women themselves that, given the understanding and information they need, they can and should be able to reduce and eradicate the symptoms themselves.

Hallelujah! And good luck!

Useful Addresses and Further Reading

UK

Angela Kilmartin
75 Mortimer Road
London N1 5AR

British Nutrition Foundation
15, Belgrave Square
London SW1X 8PS

National Action on Incontinence
4, St Pancras Way
London NW1 0PE

National Society for Research
 into Allergy
PO Box 45
Hinckley
Leics LE10 1JY

Women's Nutritional Advisory
 Service
PO Box 268
Lewes
East Sussex BN7 2QN

US

Bladder Health Council
300 West Pratt Street
Suite 401
Baltimore, MD 21201

Interstitial Cystitis Foundation
PO Box 1553
Madison Square Station
New York, NY 10159

The Simon Foundation for
 Continence
PO Box 835
Wilmette, IL 60091

All the following books are very informative and easy to read. They are available from bookshops (they should already be on the shelves or you can order them); some can also be found in pharmacies and supermarkets. My video is available by mail order (see address below).

Dr Lyle Breitkopf and Marion Bakoulis, *Endometriosis* (Thorsons)

Leon Chaitow, *Candida Albicans* (Thorsons)

Wendy Cooper, *No Change* (Arrow Books)

– *Understanding Osteoporosis* (Arrow Books)

Dr William Crook, *Are You Allergic?: Chronic Fatigue Syndrome and the yeast connection* (Professional Books)

Dr Katharina Dalton, *PMS: The Complete Guide to Treatments* (Thorsons)

Jeremy Hamand, *Prostate Problems* (Thorsons)

Philippa Harknett, *Herpes* (Thorsons)

Angela Kilmartin, *Sexual Cystitis* (Arrow Books)

Dr Richard Millard, *Overcoming Incontinence* (Thorsons)

Felicity Smart and Professor Stuart Campbell, *Fibroids* (Thorsons)

Dr Mike Smith, *Handbook of Over-the-counter Medicines* (Kyle Cathie)

–, *Handbook of Prescription Medicines* (Kyle Cathie)

–, 'Postbag Series' on *Allergies, Arthritis, Back Pain, Eating Disorders, HRT, Migraine, Skin Problems* and *Stress* (Kyle Cathie)

Shirley Trickett, *Coming Off Tranquillizers and Sleeping Pills* (Thorsons)

– *Coping Successfully with Candida* (Thorsons)

–, *The Essential Candida Abicans Cookbook* (Thorsons)

–, *Irritable Bowel Syndrome and Diverticulosis* (Thorsons)

Patsy Westcott, *Pelvic Inflammatory Disease* (Thorsons)

–, *Hormone Replacement Therapy* (Thorsons)

Overcoming Cystitis (video available from Kilmartin Videos, PO Box 217, Walton on Thames, KT12 3YF)

INDEX